MRCGP: Approaching the Modular Examination 2nd Edition

Edited and compiled by

John Sandars
MBChB(Hons) MSc FRCGP MRCP(UK)
Diploma in Counselling Diploma in Palliative Medicine
Certificate in Education
General Practitioner
Wilmslow Road Medical Centre
Handforth, Cheshire
and
Lecturer
School of Primary Care and Evidence for Population
Health Unit, University of Manchester
Manchester

Louise Newson
BSc(Hons) MBChB(Hons) MRCP MRCGP
General Practitioner
Castle Medical Centre
Kenilworth, Warwickshire

© 2002 PASTEST Ltd
Egerton Court
Parkgate Estate
Knutsford, Cheshire
Telephone: 01565 752000

First edition 1998
Second edition 2002

ISBN 1 901198 91 X

A catalogue record for this book is available from the British Library.

The information contained within this book was obtained by the authors from reliable sources. However, while every effort has been made to ensure its accuracy, no responsibility for loss, damage or injury occasioned to any person acting or refraining from action as a result of information contained herein can be accepted by the publishers or authors.

PasTest Revision Books and Intensive Courses

PasTest has been established in the field of postgraduate medical education since 1972, providing revision books and intensive study courses for doctors preparing for their professional examinations.

Books and courses are available for the following specialties:

MRCGP, MRCP Part 1 and Part 2, MRCPCH Part 1 and Part 2, MRCS, MRCOG, DRCOG, MRCPsych, DCH, FRCA and PLAB.

For further details contact:

PasTest, Freepost, Knutsford, Cheshire WA16 7BR
Tel: 01565 752000   Fax: 01565 650264
Email: enquiries@pastest.co.uk   Web site: www.pastest.co.uk

Typeset by Breeze Ltd, Manchester.
Printed by MFP Limited.

CONTRIBUTORS

Peter Acheson MbChB MRCGP DRCOG
General Practitioner (Principal)
Claremont Medical Centre
Exmouth Health Centre
Claremont Grove
Exmouth

Dr Tim Ballard FRCGP
General Practitioner
Shalbourne
Wiltshire

Sean P Coughlin MBChB MMedSc FRCGP
General Practitioner
Health Centre
Raikes Road
Great Eccleston
Preston

Dr R Daniels MA MRCGP
General Practitioner
Townsend House Medical Centre
Seaton
Devon

Dr Anwar A Khan BSc MBBS DRCOG DCH (Lond) DCCH (Edin) FRCGP
GP Trainer and Course Organiser
Loughton Health Centre
Loughton
Essex

and

Examiner
Royal College of General Practitioners
14 Princes Gate
Hyde Park
London SW7 1PU

Dr David Whillier MSc FRCGP
GP Trainer, MRCGP Examiner, MAP Assessor, Clinical Governance Lead
Woodlands Health Centre
Paddock Wood
Tonbridge
Kent TN12 6AX

PERMISSIONS

PasTest would like to thank the BMJ Publishing Group for their kind permission to reproduce extracts from the following articles:

Baxter et al. 'A cost effective community based heart health promotion project in England: Prospective Comparative Study'. BMJ 1997; 315: 582.

Dey, Collins, Woodman. 'Randomised controlled trial assessing effectiveness of health education leaflets in reducing incidence of sunburn'. BMJ 1995; 311: 1062.

Gussekloo, R G et al. 'Impact of mild cognitive impairment on survival in very elderly people: cohort study'. BMJ 1997;315:1053–4

J Kai. 'Parents' difficulties and information needs in coping with acute illness in preschool children: a qualitative study'. BMJ 1996; 313: 987–990.

Lowy et al. 'Is histological examination of tissue removed by GPs always necessary? Before and after comparison of detection rates of serious skin lesions'. BMJ 1997; 315: 406.

McDonald et al. 'Opening Pandora's Box: the unpredictability of reassurance by a normal test'. BMJ 1996; 313: 329.

Ridsdale L et al. 'Feasibility and effects of nurse-run clinics for patients with epilepsy in General Practice: randomised controlled trial'. BMJ 1997;314:120–2

Sonke GS et al. 'Comparison of case fatality in smokers and non-smokers after acute cardiac event'. BMJ 1997;315:992–3

Walma et al. 'Withdrawal of long-term diuretic medications in elderly patients: a double blind trial'. BMJ 1997; 315: 464.

Watkins J. 'Effectiveness of influenza vaccination policy at targeting patients at high risk of complications during winter 1994–5: cross sectional survey'. BMJ: 1997;315:1069–70

PasTest would also like to thank the Royal College of General Practitioners for their kind permission to reproduce the questions from their 2002 regulations.

CONTENTS

Contributor's list	iii
Permissions	iv
Preface	vi
Introduction to the MRCGP examination	vii
Revision Planning	xv

Approach to Critical Appraisal type questions — 1

Approach to Current Awareness type questions — 67

Approach to Problem solving type questions — 77

Approach to Multiple Choice type and Computer Marked questions — 105

Approach to the Oral Examination Component — 205

Approach to the Assessment of Consulting Skills component – Video — 215

Approach to the Assessment of Consulting Skills component – Simulated Surgery — 227

Approach to Membership by Assessment (MAP) — 237

Summative Assessment — 253

Passing the MRCGP: A Registrar's View — 267

Appendix 1:	The Consultation	271
Appendix 2:	Medical Audit	275
Appendix 3:	Evidence-based Medicine	277
Appendix 4:	Ethical Problem Solving	279

Recommended Reading List — 284

Multiple Choice type Question Index — 285

PREFACE

This book is not a textbook of General Practice, nor is it a last minute examination crammer. It offers a systematic approach to the MRCGP examination, providing the candidate with an invaluable insight into what the examiners are looking for and how to answer questions in order to gain the maximum marks. Several practice papers with answers are provided to help in this process.

The Royal College is constantly trying to improve the validity and reliability of the examination and minor changes may be introduced. Every effort has been made to ensure that this new book contains the most up to date information that is currently available.

This new edition would not have been possible without the help of several MRCGP examiners, General Practitioners and the members of the Examination Department.

Peter Acheson	Multiple Choice questions
Elizabeth Acheson	Multiple Choice questions
Tim Ballard	Simulated Surgery chapter
Sean Coughlin	Current Awareness type questions and Summative Assessment chapter
Rob Daniels	Multiple Choice questions
Nick Foster	Critical Appraisal type questions
Moya Kelly	Problem-solving type questions
Anwar Khan	Multiple Choice questions
Paul Middleton	Critical Appraisal type questions
Val Wass	Oral Examination chapter
David Whillier	Membership by Assessment chapter

Finally we would like to thank the publishing department at PasTest, since without their help the book would never have reached publication!

We hope that you find this book helpful and we wish you every success – not just in the MRCGP examination but in your future of General Practice.

John Sandars
Louise Newson

INTRODUCTION TO THE MRCGP EXAMINATION

The MRCGP examination has constantly evolved since it was first developed in 1965. The examination is set by the Royal College of General Practitioners as an 'assessment of the knowledge, skills and attitudes appropriate to the General Practitioner on completion of vocational training, assessing the competence of candidates to carry out unsupervised responsibility for the care of patients in General Practice'. The college expects that in the future it will be usual for the MRCGP qualification to be held by all new principals entering General Practice. The MRCGP examination is often regarded as an end-point assessment for General Practice for those completing their vocational training.

Around 2000 candidates enter the examination each year. The pass rate is approximately 70% (higher than other postgraduate exams); however the MRCGP exam cannot be described as easy and should therefore not be taken lightly.

The Structure of the Examination

The MRCGP exam is now modular, using a credit accumulation system. The main features of this new style examination are as follows:

1. Candidates must pass all four modules in order to pass the examination overall.
2. The modules may be taken at the same session, or at different sessions, and in any order. For example, candidates do not now have to pass the written papers before taking the oral.
3. Candidates may have up to two further attempts at each module (on payment of a supplementary fee in each instance).
4. All modules must be passed within three years of acceptance of the application, otherwise the entire examination has to be retaken.

The four modules of the examination are:

- Paper 1 (examiner marked)
- Paper 2 (machine marked)
- An assessment of consulting skills
- Oral examination

Each module is available twice a year, in the summer and the winter.

Paper 1 and Paper 2

The two written papers are held on the same day for the convenience of those candidates who want to take both papers at the same session, but can be taken or retaken singly. Paper 1 is held in the morning and Paper 2 in the afternoon.

Consulting Skills

Consulting skills are assessed by one of two methods:

1. A video recording of the candidate consulting with patients who have given their consent to be recorded.
2. The candidate takes part in a 'simulated surgery' in which the candidate consults with a sequence of actors who play the part of patients.

Video recording is the normal method of assessing consulting skills for the MRCGP and the simulated surgery is available only to those candidates who, in the opinion of the examiners, have insuperable difficulties in making video recordings, for example if the candidate is practising in an area where most consultations are conducted in a language other than English. Special application has to be made to the Examinations Department when a simulated surgery is requested (see later chapter).

The Oral Examination
Candidates are assigned to a centre, either London or Edinburgh, for an oral examination. This is held six to eight weeks after the written papers.

Application for the MRCGP Examination
Those doctors eligible to be an independent practitioner of General Practice or those undergoing vocational training will be allowed to sit the exam. All candidates must provide evidence of proficiency in basic cardiopulmonary resuscitation and child health surveillance at the time of application for the examination. There are other eligibility criteria, such as the length of time in practice and appropriate experience. Full details are available from the **Examinations Department, Royal College of General Practitioners, 14 Prince's Gate, Hyde Park, London, SW7 1PU (e-mail: exams@rcgp.org.uk).**

Content of the Examination

Every General Practitioner is required to have a breadth of knowledge and skills rather than large amounts of in-depth knowledge about small topics – this is the realm of the specialist. The MRCGP examination reflects this requirement and the content has no strictly defined curriculum but it sets out to test all of those areas which comprise good General Practice in the British National Health Service today. Candidates who practise within a different system of health care should be aware of this British focus and will need to be prepared appropriately.

The examination overall is designed to test the **domains of competence** required of a contemporary General Practitioner and also the various **roles** which a doctor may be required to adopt in the course of ordinary General Practice.

The Domains of Competence

- Factual knowledge
- Evolving knowledge – 'hot topics', qualitative research
- The evidence base of practice – knowledge of literature, quantitative research
- Critical appraisal skills – interpretation of literature, principles of statistics
- Application of knowledge – problem solving, clinical decision making, audit
- Personal care – matching principles to individual patients
- Written communication
- Verbal communication – the consultation process
- The practice context – practice management business skills, team issues
- The regulatory framework of practice – medico-political, legal and societal issues
- Ethnic and transcultural issues
- Values and attitudes – ethics, integrity, consistency
- Self-awareness – insight, 'the doctor as a person', reflective learning
- Commitment to maintaining standards – personal and professional growth, continuing medical education
- Problem solving – general applications, case-specific, clinical management

The various roles the doctor may adopt:

- Clinician and family physician
- The patient's advocate
- Resource allocator and gatekeeper
- Team leader and team member
- Partner and colleague
- Employer, manager and business person
- Teacher
- Researcher and learner
- Member of a profession
- Reflective practitioner
- Individual person

The wide range of knowledge – the breadth of General Practice – can be appreciated by considering the Five Areas of General Practice, which are found on page xvi. Each module of the examination is specifically designed to assess the candidate's performance in both the domains of competence and the role of the General Practitioner.

Paper 1

Paper 1 is a three and a half hour written paper which is marked by a group of examiners. Typically Paper 1 consists of 12 questions and each question makes an equal contribution to the result. Candidates will be given a combined question and answer book with one page for each question and answers are to be written on the same sheet. Candidates will be expected to give legible and concise answers but short note form is acceptable. Occasionally candidates will be required to give structured short answers in which the response is entered into a table or similar fixed format.

The completed booklet is split up and each page is sent to a different examiner. Candidates are therefore advised to answer each question independently, even if this involves repetition of part of an earlier answer.

There are four main types of questions:

1. Questions designed to test knowledge and interpretation of
    General Practice literature. The questions will normally take the

form of a direct instruction to discuss and/or evaluate the current views on a topic and the general evidence on which they are based.

The approach to this type of question is described in the section 'Approach to current awareness type questions.'

2. Questions which test the candidate's ability to evaluate and interpret written material. This material may be in the form of published papers or extracts from papers, such as summaries or methods and results sections on their own. It may also include meta-analyses, structured summaries, leading articles from journals or systematic reviews.

The approach to this type of question is outlined in the section 'Approach to critical appraisal type questions.'

3. Questions which examine the candidate's ability to integrate and apply theoretical knowledge and professional values within the setting of primary health care in the United Kingdom. These questions test the candidate's practical approach to General Practice problems and marks are gained for the management of the problem rather than for the factual knowledge.

The approach to this type of question is described in the section 'Approach to problem solving type questions.'

4. New question formats. Other question formats may appear from time to time. This is part of the naturally evolving process of ensuring that the examination is both valid (i.e. measuring what it hopes to measure) and reliable (i.e. that it measures consistently).

Paper 2

This paper is designed to test the candidate's knowledge about General Practice, both established and recent knowledge. A multiple choice question format provides an ideal method of assessing a candidate's knowledge base; and the application of this knowledge can be assessed by problem solving and extended matching type questions. Answers are recorded on machine marked sheets.

The approach to this type of question is contained in the section 'Approach to multiple choice and computer marked questions.'

Oral Examination

This consists of two consecutive oral examinations, each lasting 20 minutes and each conducted by two different pairs of examiners. This part of the examination assesses the candidate's decision-making ability, and the professional values underpinning it.

The approach to this section is outlined in 'Approach to the oral examination component.'

Assessment of Consulting Skills

Candidates are expected to submit evidence of competence in consulting skills in the form of a video recording of a sample of their recent consultations, accompanied by a completed workbook. The work book contains a videotape log, consultation assessment forms and detailed evaluation forms. Alternatively, candidates can take part in a simulated surgery.

Further details of both of these methods can be found in the section 'Approach to the assessment of consulting skills component – video' and 'Approach to the assessment of consulting skills component – simulated surgery.'

The Results

The result in each of the four modules will be reported as fail, pass or pass with merit. Approximately 25% of candidates scoring the highest marks in each module will be given a pass with merit for that module. To achieve a pass in the MRCGP examination overall, candidates must achieve at least a pass in all four modules within three years of the acceptance of the application. If this is not achieved the candidate will be deemed to have failed the examination as a whole.

Candidates can be awarded an overall pass with merit and it is possible to be awarded an overall pass with distinction. The various rules regarding the attempts allowed at each module and how the overall result is calculated can be obtained directly from the Examination Department of the Royal College of General Practitioners. The results are published on the college website as well as being sent to individual candidates.

The Examinations Department has a specific site on the college website (www.rcgp.org.uk). This site provides an invaluable free guide to the current regulations and also features samples of both Paper 1 and Paper 2 questions. There is also a commentary from the examiners that describes what they are looking for!

THE FIVE AREAS OF GENERAL PRACTICE

The MRCGP exam syllabus covers a great breadth of knowledge and the exam itself aims to measure knowledge, skills and attitudes within the Five Areas of General Practice.

1. Clinical practice – Health and disease

The candidate will be required to demonstrate knowledge of the diagnosis, management and, where appropriate, the prevention of diseases of importance in General Practice. This area includes:

- The range of normality
- The patterns of illness
- The natural history of diseases
- Prevention
- Early diagnosis
- Diagnostic methods and techniques
- Management and treatment

2. Clinical practice – Human development

The candidate will be expected to possess knowledge of human development and be able to demonstrate the value of this knowledge in the diagnosis and management of patients in General Practice. This area includes:

- Genetics
- Foetal development
- Physical development in childhood, maturity and ageing
- Intellectual development in childhood, maturity and ageing
- Emotional development in childhood, maturity and ageing
- The range of normality

3. Clinical practice – Human behaviour

The candidate must demonstrate an understanding of human behaviour, particularly as it affects the presentation and management of disease. This area includes:

- Behaviour presenting to the General Practitioner
- Behaviour in interpersonal relationships
- Behaviour of the family
- Behaviour in the doctor-patient relationship

4. Medicine and society

The candidate must be familiar with the common sociological and epidemiological concepts and their relevance to medical care and must be able to demonstrate knowledge of the organisation of medical and related services in the United Kingdom and abroad. This area includes:

- Sociological aspects of health and illness
- The uses of epidemiology
- The organisation of medical care in the UK – comparisons with other countries
- The relationship of medical services to other institutions of society

5. The practice

The candidate must demonstrate knowledge of practice organisation and administration and must be able to critically discuss recent developments in the evolution of General Practice. This area includes:

- Practice management
- The team
- Financial matters
- Premises and equipment
- Medical records
- Medico-legal matters
- Research

REVISION PLANNING

An essential part of the preparation for the exam is to develop skills which will last throughout your career. There is no substitute for good, methodical preparation for the exam, which will in turn lead to a successful result.

The most important point to remember is that this is an exam about **current General Practice** and your reading needs to reflect this. Subjects such as General Medicine, Obstetrics, Paediatrics, etc are included but they only make up a small proportion. In order to put this in perspective, it is helpful to look carefully at the Five Areas of General Practice on the preceding pages. You can see from this that:

Area 1: Health and Disease encompasses most of the areas covered in finals and found in textbooks.

Area 2: Human Development covers Paediatrics but also includes knowledge of the elderly.

Area 3: Human Behaviour is an important area in General Practice. It covers such areas as: why patients present, consultation models, the doctor-patient relationship and interpersonal relationships as they affect patients, their families and us.

Area 4: Medicine and Society covers the epidemiology and sociology of health care e.g. knowledge of the cause of disease (for example cholesterol and CHD risk). This is vital to our methods of treating such disease. This area includes the organisation of health care – a subject that has been affecting all of us recently.

Area 5: The Practice includes knowledge of practice management e.g. finances, records, premises, etc. It also includes general management skills such as delegation, time management and team development.

Covering all these areas in your revision will give you the broad knowledge-base required for the exam and for life as a GP (which is, of course, what the exam is designed to do!).

At first glance, the amount of work required can seem immense but by working through the different areas logically you will see that you already have a lot of the knowledge required. Your revision plan needs to be designed to fill the gaps. You won't fail for not understanding the cost-rent scheme (although you should know how to find out about it). You may, however, be on shaky ground if you know nothing about the management of a practice.

It is also important to remember that the exam reflects *current* practice and *current* research, not out-of-date books.

Bearing all this in mind, how can you start to cover the material?

Textbooks
You may need to read selected textbooks to cover areas in which your knowledge is deficient e.g. on the doctor-patient relationship or practice management. If you feel that you are lacking in basic medical knowledge, it may be worth reading a textbook but bear in mind all the other areas of knowledge as well. It is worth reading something on the common diseases in General Practice.

Journals
These cover the current research in General Practice. The British Journal of General Practice and BMJ are essential reading, preferably for the 12–18 months up to the exam. This task may seem daunting – but can actually be very interesting! You don't need to read everything. It is worth keeping notes on what you have read as it is useful to be able to review them as the exam date approaches. Look especially for review articles and recurrent 'topical' themes.

Reading one of the weekly newspapers, such as *Doctor, Pulse* or *General Practitioner* can give a good overview of current developments in General Practice. This can be especially useful for the viva examination.

Internet
There are numerous useful websites for GPs and Registrars. Some of the more useful ones are listed in the bibliography.

Occasional Papers and Reports from General Practice
These are the current literature of General Practice and hence include some vital reading. It is worth being aware of recent publications, as these are often clues to current areas of importance in General Practice.

As the amount of work can seem overwhelming, the best approach is to divide up the list between a group of people and ask each person to produce a short summary (i.e. 1–3 typed A4 sheets) on the paper or report which can then be shared.

Current Affairs
Newspapers, television and radio will keep you up to date and aware of current issues. The media often present subjects from a different perspective which can be useful.

Hot Topics
Paradoxically, most of these have been around for some time and again it is a matter of broad reading and being aware of current initiatives to make sure of covering them. A checklist is included to make sure you have not missed any major areas. An excellent up-to-date book '*Hot Topics for MRCGP and General Practitioners*' by L Newson and A Patel is recommended as it provides referenced overviews of various clinical and non-clinical subjects (see Appendix 5).

Courses
There are various courses designed to prepare candidates for the exam, some of them can be invaluable and can help to direct your revision and provide some very useful material for the exam.

Planning
Go through the 'five areas' and the list of revision topics to identify a list of areas on which you want to concentrate. Start with those areas you know nothing about and, if there is time, come back to topics you know better. That way you will ensure a broad knowledge base.

Ideally, get together with other people taking the exam and share out topics and Occasional Papers to produce short summaries of each. When you read a topic, try to think about the sort of questions you could be asked, e.g. managing a diabetic who will not accept the disease. Always think about the ethical issues. Remember, the difficult problems that arise in surgery are often the same ones that appear in the exam.

Practising
Practising the different components of the exam will improve your technique and help identify weak areas of knowledge.

Outside Interests

It is important not to let your life suffer when preparing for the exam. Having interests outside medicine makes you less stressed and more likely to survive!

Remember:

- Doing, discussing and communicating are as important as sitting in a room reading
- Use your patients to direct your revision
- Have an overall plan. Keep records of what you read as this helps revision and allows you to see progress from your efforts.
- Take an interest in developments within your practice throughout your training
- Steady reading throughout the year is better than pre-exam panic

Good luck!

APPROACH TO CRITICAL APPRAISAL TYPE QUESTIONS

Increasingly all General Practitioners are being faced with an array of material which has to be evaluated and interpreted. This component is found in both Paper 1 and Paper 2 and questions are designed to test the candidate's ability to:

- Analyse and interpret an audit, consider change and apply these principles to real life situations
- Critically appraise presented material. This includes an ability to state the main types of design and methodology, to recognise the strengths and weaknesses of each, to identify the sources of bias and the effects made to eliminate bias, including questionnaires, and to identify the validity and reliability of studies.
- Interpret the results of presented material. This includes knowledge of power of studies, p values, confidence intervals, NNT (numbers needed to treat), odds ratios, sensitivity, specificity and predictive values.
- Apply the strength of evidence to a clinical scenario
- Critically appraise systematic reviews, meta analyses, cost effectiveness evaluations and guidelines
- Apply an evidence-based medicine approach to a clinical scenario including formulation of a question, search strategy, appraisal of evidence and application of evidence to the clinical problem

How to Approach Critical Appraisal Questions

Critically appraising a clinical paper can seem a daunting prospect. However, like most of the things, a planned approach will make it easier.

The scope of this section is vast and only the basic principles are outlined here. Further details can be obtained by reference to the two excellent texts referred to in the recommended reading list: *How to Read a Paper* by Trisha Greenhalgh and *The Pocket Guide to Critical Appraisal* by Iain Crombie.

Critical appraisal skills are used to assess the quality of research and evidence which should underpin our clinical decision making. Critical appraisal skills concentrate on two areas:

- Basic Study Design
- Basic Statistical Interpretation

1. Basic Study Design

Typical study designs include:

Cross Sectional Study – a survey of the frequency of the disease or the risk factor in a defined population at a given time. This can assess prevalence and may generate hypotheses about associations between risk factors and diseases, but it cannot evaluate hypotheses since it does not take into account how exposure to a risk factor relates to the development of the disease.

Cohort Study – a type of observational study of a group of subjects with a specific disease or characteristic who are followed up over a period of time to detect complications or new events. This group may be compared with a control group. Often this type of study requires follow-up over several years, and it may be prone to loss of subjects and recall bias.

Case Control Study – a type of observational study in which the characteristics of subjects with a disease are compared with a selected group of control subjects without the disease. The validity of this type of study depends on the appropriate selection of control subjects.

Controlled Trial – an experimental study in which an intervention is applied to one group of subjects and the outcome compared with that in a control group who received another intervention, which may be active treatment or a placebo. Ideally patients should be assigned to treatment groups in a randomised manner. The randomised control trial is considered to be the 'gold standard'.

2. Basic Statistical Interpretation

Statistical tests can appear to be very complicated but the underlying principle to note is that these tests are used to quantify the likelihood that the observed result is a real effect rather than having arisen by chance.

There are several well recognised statistical tests that can be applied to data but detailed consideration of these is beyond the scope of this book. However, all of these tests are designed to assess the probability that observed differences could have risen purely by chance rather than through the intervention. Such tests of significance are discussed in the later glossary of terms.

An Approach to Qualitative Research

Qualitative research is often described as 'research without numbers' and this often implies that it lacks a degree of rigour. Qualitative research methods aim to understand what things mean to people and are particularly useful in defining preliminary questions for a research focus and in understanding the patient perspective. The importance of this approach is demonstrated by the increasing appearance of this type of research in medical journals.

The process of carrying out qualitative research can be divided into two broad types of activity: gathering data and analysing data.

1. Gathering qualitative data
There is a wide range of methods, including:
* Semi-structured interviews
* Participant observation
* Document research
* Focus groups
The main feature is that a 'richness' of understanding of the person's experience is obtained. This is often achieved by combining several of the above methods.

2. Analysing qualitative data
The researcher is faced with a large amount of material from which some degree of sense has to be found. This can be achieved by progression through a series of stages:
* Immersion
  The researcher intensively studies the data to 'absorb' the various meanings.
* Categorisation
  The data is systematically worked through, assigning various coding categories or themes. These can then be reduced into the core categories.
* Triangulation
  The aim of this procedure is to find agreement about the core categories. The researcher looks for convergence between the data produced from diverse sources, methods and investigators. This gives strength to the validity of the conclusion.
* Interpretation
  This involves constructing a theoretical model to explain the findings of the study.

The great strength of a qualitative approach to research is that it is possible to provide a unique snapshot into human experience.

Critical Appraisal Scheme For Clinical Trial Papers

Objectives and Hypotheses
- Can you identify clearly the objective(s) of the study?
- Do the investigators state or imply the population to which they intend to refer their findings?
- Given the above, are these important and relevant objectives?

Design of the Investigation
- Is the design of the study suitable for the proposed objectives?
- How was the sample selected? Are there possible sources of selection bias, which would make the sample atypical, and if so is a provision made to deal with this bias?
- What was the response rate and was any attempt made to assess the characteristics of non-responders?
- Was some form of control necessary, and if so is it satisfactory?
- Are inclusion and exclusion criteria for the sample clearly defined and applied?
- Is the study large enough to achieve its objectives? For numerical estimates and comparisons appropriate power calculations should be described.
- If it is a clinical trial are there clear rules for withdrawal from or stopping the trial? Is there provision for detecting likely adverse events?
- If a randomisation design is desirable has it been used and adequately described?
- If it is a multi centre trial does the organisation/co-ordination seem adequate?

Measurement and Observations
- Are there clear definitions of the terms used, including diagnostic criteria, measurements and criteria of outcome?
- Are the measurements valid, i.e. accurate?
- Are the measurements repeatable, i.e. consistent over time and between different subjects, places of measurement, etc?
- Have attempts been made to minimise bias in the measurements? If bias is clearly unavoidable has it been evaluated?

Presentation of Results
- Are the results presented clearly, objectively and in sufficient detail to enable readers to make their own judgement?
- Are the results internally consistent, i.e. do the numbers add up properly, and can the different tables be reconciled?

Analysis
- Are the data suitable for statistical analysis?
- Are the statistical methods stated and appropriate to the data?
- Are the statistical tests correctly performed and interpreted?
- Is there sufficient analysis to determine whether significant differences are in fact due to lack of comparability of the groups in age or sex, or in other relevant variables?

Discussion
- Are the results discussed in relation to existing knowledge on the subject and the study objectives?
- Is the discussion biased?

Conclusions
- Are the conclusions justified, given the methodology and results?

Style and Presentation
- Is there a clear and unambiguous style and appropriate length?
- Is the journal that the paper has been published in appropriate to the likely readership? Is it a high circulation or specialist journal?
- Are the references appropriate and up to date and relevant to the study and the conclusions?

Critical Appraisal Scheme for Review Papers
Review papers such as systematic reviews or meta-analyses are becoming increasingly common since they summarise scientific evidence on a particular topic. Such reviews save the reader from searching and appraising a whole series of articles, but this very process can lead to bias. Critical appraisal of such review papers is increasingly important since for the busy reader these reviews provide the usual scientific evidence on which clinical decisions are made.
- Did the review address a clearly focused issue, related to the population studied, the intervention given or the outcomes considered?
- Were important and relevant studies included? Has there been a wide search for published and unpublished studies, in both non-

English language and English language journals? Were appropriate databases searched and what were the search strategies?
- Have the authors of the review assessed the quality of the included studies? The quality of the review depends on the qualities of these original studies – if there are poor original studies then the review will draw inappropriate conclusions!
- Were the results similar from study to study?
- What is the overall result of the review?
- How precise are the results? Has there been statistical confirmation of precision?
- Can the results be applied to the local population? Are the patients covered by the review similar enough to the local population to which you wish to apply the results?
- Were all clinically important outcomes considered?
- Are the benefits worth the harms and costs?

Critical Appraisal Scheme for Qualitative Research Papers
- Was the research question clearly defined?
- Was a qualitative approach appropriate?
- Was the setting in which the research took place clearly described (the context)?
- Was the sampling strategy clearly defined? Sampling is designed to study the most useful or productive range of individuals and settings relevant to the research question.
- Did the researchers address the issues of subjectivity and data collection?
- Were any steps taken to increase the reliability of the data collected, for example, by using a different method or sample?
- What methods were used to analyse the data? How were themes derived from the data and how was bias reduced?
- Are the results credible and supported by the data?
- To what extent are the findings of the study transferable to other settings (generalisability)?

Critical Appraisal Scheme for Pharmaco-Economic Studies
- Have the study questions and hypothesis and design been clearly stated?
- Has the study involved a comparison of at least two alternatives? The 'do nothing', 'least-costly' and 'most-used' options should be considered.
- Have all relevant costs and benefits of the alternatives been identified and appropriately valued?

- Is the study of sufficient size to assess significant differences between alternatives?
- Have marginal costs and benefits of alternatives been valued?
- Have future costs and benefits been appropriately discounted?
- Has detailed sensitivity analysis been conducted?

Critical Appraisal Scheme for Guidelines
- Have the authors responsible for the development of the guideline been clearly identified?
- Has external funding or support been received and if so has any potential bias been taken into account?
- Are the reasons for developing the guideline clearly stated?
- Is there a description of the individuals who are involved in developing the guideline and if so did the group contain representatives of all key disciplines?
- Is there a description of the sources of information used to select the evidence on which the recommendations are based and if so are they adequate?
- Is there a description of the methods used to interpret and assess the strength of the evidence?
- How was group consensus reached?
- Is there an adequate description of the health benefits that are likely to be gained from the recommended management and is there an adequate description of the cost:benefit ratio?
- Have the guidelines been piloted and independently reviewed by experts before release?
- Is there a mention of a date for reviewing or updating the guidelines?
- Is there a mention of other sets of guidelines that deal with the same topic, and if so, is there a discussion of differences between the guidelines and reasons for them?
- Is there a satisfactory description of the patients to which the guidelines are meant to apply?
- Is there a satisfactory description of the circumstances in which exceptions may be made to using the guidelines?
- Is there an explicit statement of how patient preferences should be taken into account in applying the guidelines?
- Are the guidelines clear in describing which condition is to be detected, treated or prevented?
- Are the recommendations clearly presented?
- Do the guidelines contain a dissemination strategy and is this realistic?

- Is there a statement of how the guidelines can be adapted to local use?
- Is it possible to clearly identify standards and can the guidelines be subject to audit?

Glossary of Key Terms Used in Critical Appraisal and Basic Statistics

Bias – this refers to any methodological flaw likely to produce deviation from true observation or measurement.

- **Sample or selection bias** – in some way the sample is not representative of the population from which it comes.
- **Recall bias** – e.g. inability to recall information related to exposure to risk factors, as in case control studies.
- **Non response bias** – when information only relates to the responders, who may not be representative of the population from which the sample is drawn. Non response bias becomes less important at response rates over about 70%.

Blindness – used to describe the lack of awareness for investigators and participants of their inclusion and whether they are part of treatment or control treatment groups in order to eliminate potential bias. In single blind trials the investigator or the subject, but not both, is unaware of whether active or control therapy is being administered. In double blind trials both the investigators and the participants are unaware of allocation to control study groups.

Confidence intervals – the confidence interval (CI) is the range of values for which the observed result is compatible, i.e. the confidence interval of a result from a study sample is the range of values in which it is fairly certain that the true population value lies (usually 95%). A range of possibilities for the population value is thus estimated, giving more useful information than merely classifying the result as 'significant' or 'non significant'. If the confidence interval of the difference between treatments includes the value 0 then the study has failed to demonstrate a difference between the treatments, whereas if the value 0 is excluded from the confidence interval then a real difference is likely. Similarly, if the confidence intervals around a measure of an effect of two drugs overlap, then the study has failed to demonstrate a difference. On the other hand, if there is no overlap then a real difference is likely. More information can be gleaned by considering the width of confidence intervals.

Confounding – in any study the significance of association between variables or differences between groups may be undermined by the operation of factors, other than those under investigation, which may themselves explain part or all of the study's observations. Confounding occurs when an estimate of the association between an exposure and disease is mixed up with the real effect of another exposure on the same disease – two exposures are being correlated. Elimination of potential confounders is an important part of study design.

Correlation – when one variable changes in a defined way in relation to a second variable, the two are said to be correlated. Correlation implies an association, not causality. The correlation coefficient is a numerical expression of the strength and direction (positive or negative) of such an association.

Frequency distribution – this describes the way in which values within a given population are distributed. A normal distribution produces a uni-modal bell shaped curve in which 95% of the area under the curve lies within the range of the mean ± 1.96 times the standard deviation and 99% of the area lies within the range of the mean ± 2.58 times the standard deviation. When data is normally distributed, parametric statistical tests may be applied to them; when they are not, non-parametric statistics are used.

Incidence rate – the occurrence of new cases of a disease or condition within a specified population and period of time, e.g. the incidence of duodenal ulcer in the adult population is approximately 1% per year (compare with prevalence).

Intention to treat analysis – this is an analysis of the results in the control and treatment groups with respect to the number of patients entering the study, rather than those completing it. By including all entrants to the study, intention to treat analysis avoids biases due to failure of compliance and admits to side-effects of therapy causing subjects to drop out from therapeutic trials. It provides an estimate of the overall benefit of therapy in the population studied.

Mean – average group of values.

Median – the middle score of a group of values, i.e. the value with equal numbers of other values above and below it.

Meta-analysis – a method of analysing data from more than one study, with the theoretical advantage of increasing sample sizes. Meta-analysis may detect differences which were not apparent with any confidence in individual studies with small sample sizes. Rigorous criteria for inclusion of data into meta-analyses must be applied to ensure that the data analysed are compatible.

Mode – the most frequently occurring value in a group of values.

Null hypothesis – this is an important concept in the design of trials and the understanding of probability. Tests of significance (hypothesis testing) are carried out to assess the probability that the observed differences between treatments could have arisen purely by chance and this is done by testing the results against a 'null hypothesis' of no true difference between treatments. The result of the test is expressed as a probability, the 'p' value, of whether the observed data are consistent with the null hypothesis. By an arbitrary convention, a 'p' value below 0.05 (which represents a 1 in 20 chance) is accepted as evidence of a true difference and is described as 'significant'. Conversely 'p' values of 0.05 are regarded as being non-significant. This approach has two obvious drawbacks. Firstly, two values may be very similar e.g. $p = 0.051$ and $p = 0.049$ and although these are essentially similar values they would be regarded as non-significant and significant respectively. Secondly, significance tests give no indication of the magnitude of the observed difference between treatment, which would be more meaningful.

Odds ratio – this is the ratio of the odds of exposure among the cases, to the odds of exposure among the controls of a case control study. It is a method of expressing risk reduction, see under risk reduction measurements.

Power – power calculations involve the determination of sample sizes required to detect effect at the desired level of significance.

Predictive value – in evaluating a diagnostic test, e.g. screening, the positive predictive value is the probability of the person having the disease when the test is positive and the negative predictive value is the probability of the person not having the disease when the test is negative. Predictive value depends on the sensitivity and specificity of the test and, more importantly, on the prevalence of the disease in the population being tested.

Prevalence – the proportion of cases within a specified population at a given time (compare with incidence).

Risk reduction measurements – some clinical trials are carried out to test the effect of preventative therapy on the risk of experiencing an adverse event, and the method of describing differences in risk reduction has been shown to affect how such differences are perceived. Study results are often presented in terms of the relative risk reduction but this may give the reader a misleading impression of the actual magnitude of the benefit therapy since it does not indicate the underlying incidence of an event being prevented. The relative risk is a ratio of the incidence of disease in exposed persons to the incidence in non-exposed persons. A more useful expression of results is the NNT – number needed to treat. This is the number of patients who would need to be treated to prevent one clinical event and it is the reciprocal of the absolute risk reduction. Thus results are put in a more meaningful context, enabling comparisons between different interventions to be made. For example, the reduction in relative risk may be the same but the number needed to treat may be 20 patients in one example and 200 in another.

Sensitivity and specificity – these are terms applied to a diagnostic test, such as a screening test. A screening test must be reliable, providing consistent results, and valid, correctly categorising people into groups with or without disease. Sensitivity is the proportion of truly ill people in the screened population who are identified as ill by the screening test (probability of a positive test in people with the disease) and specificity is the proportion of truly healthy people who are so identified by the screening test (probability of a negative test in people without the disease).

Stratification – a sampling method in which individuals for study are selected from within sub-groups of a population rather than sampling from the entire population. Stratification is carried out to ensure representiveness or exclude bias.

Type 1 error – the error, in the analysis of data, of stating that a difference or effect is present when in fact it is not. Conventionally a numerical value is often set at 0.05, i.e. on 5% of occasions the size of difference found could have occurred entirely by chance.

Type 2 error – the error, in the analysis of data, of concluding that a difference or effect is not present when in fact it is – this is particularly important when sample sizes are small.

CRITICAL APPRAISAL SAMPLE QUESTIONS (A)

The following four papers show the range of research papers that can appear in journals. The papers include a case control study, a cross sectional survey, a randomised trial and a cohort study. Each study method has specific reasons for its use, according to the strength of evidence it presents as well as how it is interpreted and what precautions are needed in interpretation.

These sample questions will provide important practice on doing critical appraisal. The principles apply to the MRCGP examination but these questions are not typical of the format that you will be presented with.

The principles applying in these sample questions provide important practice on critical appraisal type questions. The MRCGP question format, however, may vary to reflect current emphasis within the exam. In your answer, restrict yourself to answering the question, and avoid widening the discussion to related topics unless asked to do so. Remember that the exercise is to see how well you can interpret a paper and understand its conclusions. In any paper, there are good and bad points contributing to how reliable and valid the interpretation is. In your answer use these points to justify your views on the strengths (and weaknesses) of the paper.

Critically appraise this article, focusing on the strengths and weaknesses of the study.

Paper reference: Sonke GS *et al.* Comparison of case fatality in smokers and non-smokers after acute cardiac event; BMJ 1997;315:992–3.

Introduction

Although smoking is a major modifiable risk factor for acute myocardial infarction, it has also been associated with an up to twofold lower risk of dying in hospital after an acute myocardial infarction. We analysed data from a community-based register of coronary heart disease to determine whether differences in case fatality (the proportion of those dying) between smokers and non-smokers are restricted to patients who have been admitted to hospital and to evaluate possible explanations for this smoker's paradox.

Subjects, methods, and results

All deaths related to coronary causes and all admitted patients aged 25–64 who met predefined criteria for myocardial infarction or coronary death were identified in Auckland, New Zealand, between 1986 and 1992 as part of the World Health Organisation MONICA (monitoring trends and determinants in cardiovascular disease) project. Study criteria, and methods of case finding and data collection procedures have been published. Post-mortem examinations were performed on 63% of those who died from cardiac causes. Deaths before admission to hospital, deaths within 28 days after admission, and the total number of deaths were measured. Smoking was determined by direct questioning of surviving patients and of relatives of those who died. Patients were classed as current smokers (those who smoked at least one cigarette a week at the onset of symptoms or gave up smoking less than one month before the index event), ex-smokers (those who had abstained from smoking for at least one month before the onset of symptoms), or non-smokers (those who had never smoked). Logistic regression models were used to assess the effects of smoking on case fatality after adjusting for age, sex, history of myocardial infarction, and history of angina. For those admitted to hospital, adjustments were based on whether they received thrombolytic treatment. An adjustment for the year of infarction was included to account for time trends in event rates.

Demographic information, case fatality, crude odds ratio, and adjusted odds ratio by smoking status for acute cardiac events in patients aged 25–64 years, 1986–92

	Non-smokers (n=1088)	Current smokers (n=2166)	Ex-smokers (n=1477)
Mean (SD) age (years)	55.8 (7.2)	53.3 (8.2)	56.7 (6.6)
No (%) men	801/1088 (73.6)	1689/2166 (78.0)	1229/1477 (83.2)
No (%) with previous myocardial infarction	257/1084 (23.7)	436/2153 (20.2)	552/1475 (37.4)
No (%) with previous angina	243/1086 (22.4)	342/2158 (15.8)	301/1476 (20.4)
Case fatality (%)			
Before admission to hospital:	409/1088 (37.6)	831/2166 (38.4)	503/1477 (34.0)
Crude odds ratio* (95% Cl) (n=4731)	1.00	1.03 (0.89 to 1.20)	0.86 (0.73 to 1.01)
Adjusted odds ratio* (95% Cl)	1.00	1.09 (0.93 to 1.27)	0.79 (0.67 to 0.94)
After admission to hospital:	123/679 (18.1)	157/1335 (11.8)	197/974 (20.2)
Crude odds ratio* (95% Cl) (n=2988)	1.00	0.60 (0.47 to 0.78)	1.13 (0.88 to 1.45)
Adjusted odds ratio* (95% Cl)	1.00	0.72 (0.55 to 0.95)	0.93 (0.71 to 1.22)
Total:	532/1088 (48.9)	988/2166 (45.6)	700/1477 (47.4)
Crude odds ratio* (95% Cl) (n=4731)	1.00	0.88 (0.76 to 1.01)	0.94 (0.81 to 1.10)
Adjusted odds ratio* (95% Cl)	1.00	0.97 (0.84 to 1.13)	0.85 (0.72 to 1.00)

*Odds ratio is the estimated odds of dying relative to a non-smoker.

Between January 1986 and December 1992, 5106 patients with a definite myocardial infarction or who died from coronary causes were identified. Of these, 2166 were current smokers, 1477 were ex-smokers, and 1088 were non-smokers; information on smoking was missing for 375 patients, 231 of whom died before admission to hospital. Smokers were younger, more likely to be men, and fewer of them had a history of coronary heart disease when compared with non-smokers (table). The ex-smokers were older, more likely to be men, and more of them had previously had a myocardial infarction when compared with non-smokers.

Compared with non-smokers, smokers had a higher risk of dying before hospital admission but this was not significant. The risk of dying after hospital admission was significantly lower in smokers. Overall, there was no significant effect of smoking on total case fatality because smokers who die before admission have a bigger effect on total case fatality than smokers who survive to be admitted. Ex-smokers had lower risks of dying both before and after hospital admission, resulting in an overall reduction in case fatality when compared with non-smokers.

Funding: Health Research Council of New Zealand and the National Heart Foundation of New Zealand.
Conflict of interest: None.

Strengths

- Clear aims: death in smokers/non-smokers after cardiac event. This is an important area of health education in reducing mortality from smoking
- Study type: case-controlled study matching the risk of dying between smokers and non-smokers following an acute myocardial infarction
- Matching: study group of smokers is matched to a control group of non-smokers
- Group selection: it is a register-based study looking at all patients in Auckland with coronary-related deaths. This reduces bias with regard to case selection.
- Size: large number of cases (5106)
- Control matching: the mean age and age standard deviation (SD) is similar in all three groups
- Endpoint: death is a well-defined specific endpoint
- Statistical analysis: a logistic regression model allows us to assess the importance of several variables simultaneously, in this case age, sex, previous heart disease and previous MI, thereby reducing the effect of confounding (the explanation of the apparent difference between the two groups is in fact due to another unmeasured factor)
- Method: study criteria, methods of case finding and data collection procedures have been published

Weaknesses

- Case control study: lies lower down in the hierarchy of evidence
- Case control study: shows association and not causation, i.e. the study does not say smoking causes less deaths following an acute cardiac event, it merely suggests an association which could equally be explained by other means
- Relevance to my practice: do patients in Auckland, New Zealand match my own patients in the UK, i.e. are the results applicable to my population
- Socio-economic data: no mention of racial characteristics and other socio-economic characteristics
- Other risk factors: no mention regarding weight, blood pressure, and cholesterol which could equally be factors relating to cardiac death
- Control matching: the three groups are not evenly matched in all aspects. A 10% difference in numbers of men between non-smokers and ex-smokers, and a 25 difference in absolute numbers between those with angina and no angina.

Critically appraise this article focusing on the strengths and weaknesses of the study.

Paper reference: Watkins J. Effectiveness of influenza vaccination policy at targeting patients at high risk of complications during winter 1994–5: cross sectional survey; BMJ: 1997;315:1069–70.

Introduction
Each year the chief medical officer writes to General Practitioners and other health professionals reminding them of the need to identify and vaccinate patients at risk of the complications of influenza – that is people who have chronic heart, chest, or kidney disease; people who have diabetes; people who are immunocompromised owing to treatment or disease; and people living in residential accommodation. Routine immunisation of elderly people is not recommended. Current data on the efficacy of influenza vaccine indicates that up to 70% of clinical cases could be prevented, an important finding as in 1989, 26,000 people, mostly elderly, or those recommended for vaccination, died in the United Kingdom from influenza and its complications. That year there was a good antigenic match between the epidemic strain and the one used in the vaccine, yet only one third to one half of all patients who would have benefited from vaccination received it. I investigated the implementation of current vaccine policy.

Subjects, methods, and results
In September 1994, 64 general practices in the county of Gwent, with a registered population of 291,908, took part in a study that entailed data collection from patients at the time of vaccination. Patients were asked their age, whether they suffered with any of the conditions for which influenza vaccination is recommended, and the method by which they came to receive vaccination. A numerical coding system was used to separate out each chronic disease and the method used to contact patients. Only practices that were computer-linked to the health authority patient register were used, and this provided patient denominator data. Practices for which the authority held denominator data on chronic diseases were used to calculate uptake rates of vaccine in at risk groups. Statistical analysis was carried out with SPSS 6.0 for Windows.

For the 28,433 doses of vaccine given in the 64 practices, information was submitted on 21,001 patients (74%). Overall, the vaccine uptake rate was 97.4 doses/1000 patients (table), though individual practices showed wide variation (range 25/1000 to 275/1000). Uptake rates in specific at-risk groups were calculated for the practices that had recorded all of their immunisations. Analysis showed that under half of those patients identified as high risk and recommended for vaccination received it: only 63% of patients with heart disease, 39% with diabetes, 41% with asthma, and only one in three of those over 75. One quarter of all doses were given to patients at low risk. The table shows that advice from General Practitioners accounted for 40% of all those being vaccinated, most of the remainder resulting from self-referral by patients on an annual basis or on advice from the practice nurse. Other health professionals, particularly hospital consultants, played an insignificant part in vaccine promotion. Under 4% of patients were recruited by proactive methods such as telephone, letter, or a message on repeat prescriptions; 80% were recruited opportunistically. Poster campaigns had little influence in targeting those who would most benefit. There was no significant difference in uptake rates between practices according to whether they were training practices or fundholders, had more than two partners, or occupied cost-rent premises. There was also no relation with list size, though those practices with the highest vaccination rates had the highest uptake in those who would most benefit.

Doses of influenza vaccine given to patients at high and low risk, showing relation with methods by which patients were contacted. Numbers in parentheses are percentages of total doses arising from that method of contact, unless stated otherwise.

Contact method	Patients of all ages at high risk	Well patients <65 years at low risk	Well patients 65 years or over at low risk	Patients with other conditions not recommended for vaccination	Total doses given (% of total doses given to study population)
Advice from General Practitioner	5495 (64)	480 (5.6)	1737 (20.2)	869 (10.1)	8581 (40.9)
Repeat prescription	263 (35.9)	73 (10)	332 (45.3)	64 (8.7)	732 (3.5)
Practice clinic	59 (86.7)	0	5 (7.4)	4 (5.9)	68 (0.3)
Hospital consultant	42 (84)	1	1	6 (12)	50 (0.2)
Practice nurse	1809 (58.5)	232 (7.5)	563 (18.2)	486 (15.7)	3090 (14.8)
Health visitor	48 (46.2)	4 (3.8)	50 (48)	2	104 (0.5)
District nurse	83 (53.5)	7 (4.5)	43 (27.7)	22 (14.2)	155 (0.7)
Postal reminder	77 (70.6)	3	28 (25.7)	1	109 (0.5)
Telephone reminder	54 (66.6)	9 (11.1)	8 (9.8)	10 (12.3)	81(0.4)
Poster in surgery	243 (38.6)	153 (24.3)	72 (11.4)	161 (25.6)	629 (3)
Awareness due to media	66 (34.5)	63 (33)	27 (14.1)	35 (18.3)	191 (0.9)
Receive vaccine each year	2168 (40.9)	1079 (20.3)	1445 (27.2)	608 (11.5)	5300 (25.2)
Other methods	476 (24.9)	691 (36)	408 (21.3)	336 (17.5)	1911 (9)
Total (% of total doses given to study population)	10883 (51.8)	2795 (13.3)	4719 (22.5)	2604) (12.4	21001 (100)

Funding: The study was made possible by a research grant from the Association for Influenza Monitoring and Surveillance.
Conflict of interest: None

Strengths

- Clear aims: influenza vaccination targeted at the 'at risk' groups
- Study importance: important area with high morbidity (26,000 people died in 1989). 70% of deaths could be prevented
- Study type: cross sectional survey appropriate for aim of study. Such a study looks to see how things are now, at a given point in time. Data is collected at a single point in time.
- Study groups: well accepted risk groups identified (those patients with heart, lung, kidney disease, diabetes and immunocompromised, as well as those in residential institutions)
- Study size: large population studied

- Question objectives: target group (patients in General Practice) fulfils Health Service managers' objectives

Weaknesses

- Paper clarity: there is lack of clarity in the paper. Figures seem to be mentioned without reference to tables. The figures are presented as fact without reference to result data
- Non-responders: large non-response rate (26%)
- Results: large skew with possible non-parametric data. Large variation from practice to practice (uptake rate 25/1000 to 275/1000). The average uptake rate of 97.4/1000 shows that more practices are at the lower limit than the higher limit. Due to the large skew in practice response rate, potential spurious and misleading estimates of significance can occur. Interestingly, there is no mention of result significance.
- Questionnaire setting: as the study was done in a General Practice setting, it is not surprising that 40.9% of patients recorded that their vaccination was a result of advice given by their GP. May have had a different result from asking patients in a hospital setting.
- Health authority data accuracy: data depends on practice database; notoriously unreliable. The chronic disease database held by the FHSA only shows those patients with asthma, and not those with chronic chest disease hence an overestimate of influenza vaccine uptake due to denominator database problems
- Database source: Unclear as to how many of the 64 practices were involved in the final study

Critically appraise this article, focusing on the strengths and weaknesses of the study.

Paper reference: Ridsdale L *et al*; Feasibility and effects of nurse-run clinics for patients with epilepsy in General Practice: randomised controlled trial; BMJ 1997;314:120–2.

Introduction
Self-help groups, such as the British Epilepsy Association, have identified unmet needs for information and counselling among patients with epilepsy. Recognising the unmet needs of such patients, the National Society for Epilepsy adopted a model used for other chronic conditions (such as diabetes) of training nurses to help patients to manage their own condition.

We evaluated the usual care provided to 251 patients with epilepsy in six General Practices. We found that the advice which their doctors viewed as important for self-management had frequently not been provided or recorded in the patients' notes. We then aimed to test the feasibility and effect of setting up a nurse-run clinic in each of the six practices. We aimed (a) to establish whether patients with epilepsy would be willing to attend nurse-run clinics and whether this would lead to more advice and monitoring of anti-epileptic drugs and (b) to ascertain the effect of the clinics on recording of advice on specified topics related to epilepsy.

Patients and methods
The patients were all aged over 15 years, either took anti-epileptic drugs or had had a diagnosis of epilepsy and an attack in the previous two years, met specified inclusion criteria, and had responded to a question-naire on their physical and psychological condition. (The method for identifying patients is described elsewhere.)

We extracted from patients' records information on advice recorded as having been given to the 251 patients on specified topics (see table 2); this was stage 1 of the study. The patients were then randomised either to intervention (n=127) or to 'usual care' (n=124). Those in the intervention group were offered an appointment with a nurse with special training in epilepsy (DR) at what was called a neurology clinic; those in the usual care group received care from their General Practitioner or Specialist (the care is described elsewhere).

The nurse-run clinics took place at the patients' own practice. The first appointment was for 45–50 minutes. The nurse asked about the frequency of epilepsy attacks and how patients managed their drugs; she took a blood sample for determination of plasma concentration of the drug if the patient was taking phenytoin, phenobarbitone, or carbamazepine and had not had the concentration determined in the past year. Individual concerns were discussed. She also gave advice on various medical and social aspects of epilepsy when appropriate, together with information leaflets. The nurse used a structured record card to record the advice she gave.

A second appointment lasting 15–20 minutes was offered three months later. At this visit drug concentrations and drug taking were reviewed and advice and support offered. The nurse again used a structured record card to record the advice she gave.

About three months after the second appointment participants were sent a second questionnaire, and advice given was reassessed using data extraction forms (stage 2). t test and x2 tests were used to make comparisons between respondents and non-respondents and between the intervention group and the group receiving usual care.

Table 1 Nurse's reported findings and proposals* for changes in drug management about which she wrote to General Practitioners of 28 patients

Finding or proposal	No of patients
Proposed referral to specialist (patient taking several drugs; poor control)	9
Proposed increased dose of anti-epileptic drugs	5
Found adverse effects from anti-epileptic drugs	4
Found mismatch between specialist advice and drug taken	3
Proposed decrease in total daily drug dose	3
Proposed clobazam before menstruation	3
Proposed reduction in frequency of drug taking (but no overall reduction)	3

*There was more than one finding or proposal for some patients.

Results

Participation and response rates have been described previously. We found no significant differences in the age, sex, or recency of seizure for the two groups. Of the 127 patients offered a first appointment with the specialist nurse, 106 (83%) attended. No significant difference was found between patients who did and did not attend in terms of age (52.1 years v 48.5 years respectively, P = 0.782) and sex (54.7% female v 52.4% male, P = 0.849). When offered a second appointment, 97/106 (92%) patients attended; 97/127 (76%) patients therefore attended both appointments. Between stage 1 and stage 2, 11 patients moved away, three died, and two were withdrawn by General Practitioners or carers because of illness that met the exclusion criteria, leaving 235 patients in the study.

Drug management
At the start of the study 169/251 (67%) patients were taking only one drug for their epilepsy. During the six months before stage 1, 36/127(29%) patients randomised to nurse-run clinics and 29/124 (23%) patients randomised to usual care had had their blood concentration checked (P = 0.28). By stage 2, 80/121 (66%) patients randomised to nurse-run clinics and 19/114(17%) patients randomised to usual care had had their blood concentration checked (P < 0.01) in the previous six months. In some cases the nurse believed that the patients' drug management might be improved, and she wrote 28 letters to patients' General Practitioners about this (table 1).

Recording clinical advice before and after intervention
Clinical data were extracted from the notes of 232 out of the original 251 patients (119/127 in the intervention group and 113/124 in the usual care group) at stage 2. Table 2 shows the results according to intention to treat, which was the offer of appointments to see the nurse. The percentage of records with advice recorded as having been given on specified topics was not significantly different at stage 1 for the two groups. At stage 2 the percentage of records with advice recorded as having been given for each topic was significantly different (P<0.000 1), with more information recorded as given in the group randomised to a nurse-run clinic.

Table 2 Advice recorded as having been given to patients receiving usual care and to patients attending nurse-run clinic. Values are numbers (percentages) of patients.

Advice	Stage 1		Stage 2	
	Usual care	Nurse-run clinic	Usual care	Nurse-run clinic
	(n=124)	(n=127)	(n=113)	(n=119)
Driving	57 (46)	59 (46)	52 (46)	84 (71)
Drug compliance	31 (25)	32 (25)	29 (26)	95 (80)
Adverse drug affects	10 (8)	13 (10)	18 (16)	86 (72)
Alcohol	13 (10)	15 (12)	16 (14)	92 (77)
Self-help groups	5 (4)	3 (2)	6 (5)	79 (66)

Strengths

- Clear aims: attendance, improving monitoring, and improving record keeping of advice
- Study criteria clearly defined: drug levels and management, advice, and recording of fit frequency
- Subject group defined: >15 yr, ± medication, epilepsy
  Inclusion criteria: answered questionnaire
- Study type: randomised control trial identifying a group of patients with epilepsy with random allocation to intervention
- Group matching: equal numbers in two groups
- Group matching: no significant differences in age, sex or recency of seizure
- Method: patient identification and usual GP care described in another paper
- Results: analysed by intention to treat, this avoids the problem of events happening to the study groups (drug dose alteration, treatment changes)

Weaknesses

- Study size: small
- Study group: the six practice demographics are not described. Are there equal numbers of patients in both arms of the study from each practice?
- Randomisation: no mention as to how the randomisation is achieved. Are all the patients randomised, or is the randomisation done within each practice?
- Nurse intervention: a nurse having 20–45 minutes to see one patient is not the same work pressure as a GP with average consultation rates. Comparability of the two study groups.
- Study implications: the study looks at process rather than management. It treats record keeping as an indicator of epilepsy management. Do poor records mean poor management?
- Patient numbers: not all patients accounted for. Started with 251 patients, 16 patients dropped out on entering stage 2 of trial (235 patients) but data extracted in Table 2 add up to 232 patients, the missing patients being in the GP arm of the study.
- Statistics: stage 2 of the trial looked at the data entered by the nurse in stage 1 of the trial. It is therefore not surprising that the records were more complete, i.e. the conclusion could have been anticipated. This is reported as highly significant (P <0.0001) with

more information recorded in the nurse-run clinic! The significance is meaningless in this context
- Study period: three months is short
- Outcome: medical outcome is not looked at, i.e. do the patients benefit medically over the long term with this extra input and time provided in the nurse-run clinic?

Critically appraise this article, focusing on the strengths and weaknesses of the study.

Paper reference: Gussekloo, R G *et al*. Impact of mild cognitive impairment on survival in very elderly people: cohort study; BMJ 1997;315:1053–4.

Introduction
Severe cognitive impairment is associated with increased mortality, but the impact of mild cognitive impairment on survival remains unclear. Although there is doubt whether a simple test such as the mini-mental state examination has sufficient discriminatory power to detect mild cognitive impairment in elderly people, we determined the impact of borderline scores in this particular examination on survival in very elderly people.

Subjects, methods, and results
As part of the Leiden 85-plus study, we followed a cohort of 891 subjects (641 women, 250 men) aged 85 years and over (median age 90 (range 85–103) years) from 1986 onwards. At entry to the study the score on the mini-mental state examination (Dutch version) was assessed by a physician during a home visit. In co-operation with the local government all but two subjects were followed for survival up to 1 October 1996. In all, 790 subjects died. Relative risks of mortality were estimated in a Cox proportional hazards model, which was adjusted for sex and for age at baseline.

During the first year of follow up, the annual mortality risk for subjects with mild cognitive impairment (score 24–27 points, n = 226) was twice as high (relative risk 1.8 (95% confidence interval 1.1–3.0)) as the annual mortality risk for subjects with a normal cognitive function (score 28–30 points, n = 352). This difference in risk remained similar until the seventh year of follow up, after which the annual mortality risk decreased to unity.

The cumulative mortality risk of the subjects with a mild cognitive impairment during the first seven years of follow up was 1.7 (1.4–2.0). This risk estimate was similar for men and women and for subjects below and over 90 years of age at baseline. Compared with subjects with a normal cognitive function, the cumulative mortality risk for subjects with a moderate cognitive impairment (score 19–23 points, n = 131) was 2.5 (2.0–3.1), and for subjects with a severe cognitive impairment (score 0–18 points, n = 180) the risk was 2.8 (2.3–3.4). The association of scores in the mini-mental state examination and mortality is further illustrated in the figure representing the survival probabilities of subjects, calculated from the age of 86 years onwards.

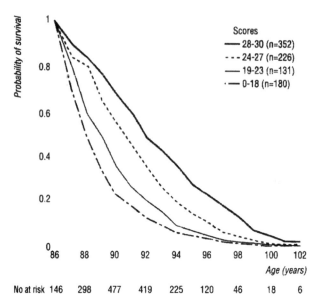

Survival probabilities from age of 86 years onwards for various categories of scores in the mini-mental state examination. Survival probabilities are calculated on data for 889 individuals followed for seven years, using an actuarial method allowing individuals to enter survival table at different years of age (left censoring)

Funding: This study was partly funded by NIH (grant 5, RO I AG 06354) and by the Ministry of Health, Welfare and Sports.
Conflict of interest: None.

Strengths

- Clear aims: mortality associated with mild cognitive impairment
- Study type: cohort study following patients through time to determine what happens to them. The design of the study is appropriate to the stated aims.
- Study period: analysis is for an appropriate length of time (7 years) with the direction of time forward (i.e. not backwards as in a retrospective study)
- Bias reduction: the analysis has tried to balance the bias of age/sex difference by using a Cox proportional hazards model. The outcome (endpoint) of death is well defined and straightforward.

- Control group: those with normal cognitive function are used for comparison, with reference to this control group
- Graph: well laid out and clear
- Study numbers: large
- Statistical results: the cumulative mortality risk during the first seven years does appear to show a true difference with the mild (1.4–2), moderate (2–3.1) and severe (2.3–3.4) confidence intervals compared with normal cognitive function. There is overlap, however, in the moderate and severe group suggesting the significance may not be all that strong in these areas.

Weaknesses

- Measurement: how accurate is mini-mental state questionnaire? Has it been validated to demonstrate levels of cognitive impairment? A full mental health questionnaire may have been more valid and powerful in defining the groups more precisely.
- Patient source: not clearly defined – the only reference is the Leiden-85 plus study. How were these 891 patients identified?
- Confounding: when an observed relationship between two variables is due to the action of a third. In this case the relationship of cognitive impairment and mortality may in fact be due to the action of a third (unaccounted for) variable such as disease. Other diseases that themselves are associated with cognitive impairment, such as cerebrovascular disease, may themselves lead to a decreased survival. In this example, it is the stroke that decreases survival rather than the reduced cognitive function
- Follow-up: no mention is made to any patients lost to follow-up. Is this because the Leiden-85 group is already a pre-selected group and therefore open to bias?
- Interview technique: when patients are being interviewed, the nature of the questioning could influence the answers obtained. It is important that the questioner asks the questions in a standard manner and in a standard way.
- Results: scoring system for cognitive impairment is not equal for all groups. The normal group had 3 scores (28–30), the mild group 4 scores (24–27), the moderate group 5 scores (19–23) and the severe group had 19 scores (0–18). How has mild been defined?
- Disease matching: this was not mentioned or allowed for between the groups

CRITICAL APPRAISAL PRACTICE QUESTIONS (B)

These questions are typical of those that you will be given in the MRCGP examination Paper 1.

QUESTION 1

Your Practice Nurse approaches you and wants to set up a 'Healthy Heart Clinic' in the Practice. She asks if you think the following study might be worth reading.

(i)   List the strengths and weaknesses of the methodology in the abstract provided.
(ii) Basing your answer on this abstract briefly describe what advice you could offer as she reads the study herself.

A cost-effective, community-based heart health promotion project in England: prospective comparative study
Paper Reference: Baxter *et al*; A cost effective community based heart health promotion project in England: Prospective Comparative Study; BMJ 1997; 315:582–6.

Reprinted with the kind permission of the *British Medical Journal*.

Introduction

Once established, coronary heart disease is impossible to cure, so a successful prevention strategy is the only way to reduce the long-term burden. Lifestyle risk factors are associated with the development of and mortality from coronary heart disease.[1-7] Prevention projects that focus on lifestyle risk factor modification have been shown to reduce the development of coronary heart disease and mortality from it.[8-11]

In 1991 we began a controlled, before and after study of the effects of a health promotion programme (Action Heart) using a population approach lasting four years to determine whether such an intervention was cost-effective in a typical non-teaching, English health district. The findings for children have been reported elsewhere.[12] We now report our findings in adults. Our objective was to evaluate the potential for producing lifestyle changes that affect the development of coronary heart disease.

Method

The study design was a prospective, comparative study of the effects of the Action Heart health promotion intervention among two populations of adults. The intervention area, the adjacent communities of Swinton and Wath, was chosen for its high incidence of coronary heart disease. The control area (Maltby) had a similar record for coronary heart disease and socio-economic composition (table 1). It was also sufficiently far from the intervention area to minimise contamination.

Action Heart used several recognised health promotion approaches[13] (see appendix 2 (www.bmj.com)).

Table 1 Standardised mortality ratios (SMR) from coronary heart disease in 1981–8 (95% confidence intervals) and rankings and values of electoral wards for deprivation indicators for control (Maltby) and intervention (Swinton and Wath) areas in 1990

Under 65 SMR 1981–1988	Maltby	Swinton	Wath
Men	138 (129–147)	131 (123–139)	136 (128–144)
Women	190 (184–196)	176 (171–181)	170 (165–175)
Deprivation rankings* (and values):			
Jarman score	14 (3.5)	12 (1.5)	9 (-1.2)
Department of the Environment index	13 (0)	11 (-0.6)	8 (-1.0)
Rotherham Metropolitan Borough Council index	16 (28)	9 (12.0)	13 (23.0)
Unemployment rate	12 (11.8)	10 (11.3)	7 (10.4)

*Among the 22 electoral wards in Rotherham

We assessed risk factor status using a self-completed questionnaire covering personal details, sources of health information, personal history of blood pressure and cholesterol measurement, family health history, diet, exercise and smoking. Questions were chosen on the basis that they had previously been used in postal questionnaires; were free from bias and ambiguity; were appropriate for the Action Heart survey; had content validity; and were the subject of previous research.[14] [15] The questions relating to smoking and milk consumption are shown in appendix 1 (www.bmj.com).

At the time of sample size determination we did not know whether our study would receive funding and whether we could do a follow-up survey. However, we wanted to have good estimates of risk factor prevalence in the populations, while recognising that the sample size would be limited by the financial resources available. In undertaking sample size calculations based on confidence interval estimates, we assumed that (a) levels of risk factors in both areas were the same at baseline; (b) reductions in the level of cigarette smoking were the primary endpoint; (c) the prevalence of smoking in both areas was 34% at baseline; and (d) reductions over three years in the prevalence of cigarette smoking attributable to Action Heart which would be considered of public health importance were of the order of 2%. To estimate smoking prevalence within 1% of the true value with 95% probability required an achieved sample size of 1,509 from each area. To attain this, we mailed 1,887 questionnaires to each area assuming an 80% response rate. We assumed that any background changes in smoking prevalence would be the same in both areas. The General Household Survey estimated that smoking prevalence was reducing by 1% per year in the age groups chosen.[16]

Questionnaires were mailed to a randomly chosen sample of named adults from the Rotherham Family Health Services Authority population age-sex register. The baseline survey was carried out in July 1991. The post-intervention survey was carried out in June 1995 using a similar approach but sent to a different random sample. (Following the cohort of individuals identified in the baseline survey would have increased statistical power but cost too much.)

The proportions of questionnaires mailed to the subgroups of men or women aged 18–40 or 41–64 were the same in both intervention and control areas for the 1991 survey. In the 1995 survey the proportions of mailed questionnaires were adjusted to try to achieve equal numbers of respondents in each of the four age-sex subgroups based on the 1991 survey response rates. This ensured best estimates of risk factor prevalences in the subgroups. However, the response proportions for age-sex subgroups were not the same as those in the underlying population for both areas as measured by the 1991 and 1995 estimates from the Office of Population Censuses and Surveys modified by local authority estimates. To adjust for over-coverage and under-coverage in the four age-sex subgroups due to this sampling frame error[17] we weighted the responses so that they were directly proportional to the corresponding subgroups in the OPCS ward populations. Weighted data were used only in the univariate analysis. Age and gender terms were used in all of the logistic regression models.

Coding – Decision rules for coding to define outcomes were made by the senior registrar in public health and a research officer.

Analysis – A univariate analysis was used to compare the prevalence of lifestyle risk factors between the control and intervention communities from 1991 to 1995. The effect of the intervention on lifestyle behaviours was evaluated using multiple logistic regression to model the proportion with a particular behaviour in the study communities as a function of age-group (18–40 or 41–64), sex, the year of observation (1991 or 1995) and area (intervention or control). After modelling the prevalence of the lifestyle behaviours for sex, area and age group separately, the effect of the intervention was measured by comparing the change in the proportion showing that behaviour between 1991 (pre-intervention) and 1995 (post-intervention) in the intervention area with the change between 1991 and 1995 in the control area, the test being based on the interaction between year and area. We also examined whether the effect of the intervention differed between the age groups and sexes.

Economics – A cost-effectiveness analysis was undertaken from the perspective of the purchaser, Rotherham Health Authority, to determine the technical efficiency of the Action Heart programme compared with traditional investment in disease management and other health promotion approaches to coronary heart disease. Outcomes were measured in units of life years gained, estimated from reported changes in smoking status using an epidemiological model. Cost data were collected in two ways. Firstly, data were extracted from financial records kept during the trial which listed actual expenditure over the four year study from a designated budget. Secondly, estimates of non-project staff costs and overheads incurred by the project were measured using diaries and timesheets kept by staff since the launch of Action Heath. Whitley Council pay scale rates were used to estimate the value of staff time. Costs relating to the research aspects of the trial were excluded from this analysis. Costs were discounted at the government recommended rate of 6%.[18]

SPECIMEN ANSWER FOR QUESTION 1

(i)
STRENGTHS
Design
- Community-based study in peer reviewed journal
- Prospective control design seems appropriate. Control group selection reasonable.

Questionnaire
- Seems thorough, and some evidence of prior reliability

Intervention
- Details of programme readily available and 'recognised' approaches used

WEAKNESSES
Sample
- Initial sample size calculated without follow-up survey even planned
- Are the assumptions made in calculating sample size valid? No justification of them
- Different cohort used in follow-up survey for financial reasons

Risk factor assessment
- Self-reporting in questionnaire – likely bias and no objective tests employed
- Weighting process used to adjust for different age-sex subgroup responses

Outcome
- Coding process not explicit
- Economic outcome measured in terms of mortality only (i.e. not morbidity)
- Analysis of changes in behaviour relies heavily on validity of projection models

(ii)
Advice to the Nurse
- Find out how far the study group is representative of her practice
- Ascertain details of exactly what the intervention involved
- Try and identify from the results any objective changes achieved and whether these can reliably be converted into long term outcomes

QUESTION 2

Your practice is considering a review of all elderly patients who are on long term diuretics to see if they can be withdrawn. You wish this approach to be evidence-based.

(i)   How would you gather the evidence?
(ii) Consider one identified study. Comment on the strengths and weaknesses of the methodology.
(iii) What conclusions can be drawn from the study?

Paper reference: Walma *et al;* 'Withdrawal of long term diuretic medications in elderly patients: a double blind trial'; BMJ 1997; 315:464.

Reprinted with the kind permission of the *British Medical Journal.*

Introduction
Diuretics are among the most frequently prescribed drugs in Western societies, with about 20% of elderly patients using them long term.[1-3] Heart failure and hypertension are the major indications, and the cost-effectiveness of diuretics in these conditions is well established. Inappropriate prescribing, however, based on premature indications or uncritical repetitions of prescriptions, leads to unnecessary use of diuretics and should be minimised because of potentially serious side-effects such as hypokalemia, hyponatraemia, dehydration, and cardiac arrest.[4-6] For the treatment of hypertension, dose reduction or cessation is generally recommended when blood pressures remain within normal limits over one to two years of treatment.[7-8] In heart failure new insights about the harmful long-term effects of chronic activation of the renin-angiotensin-aldosterone system by diuretic therapy have led to an increasing number of recommendations to aim for the lowest possible dose of diuretics.[9-11] The possibility of withdrawing diuretic therapy in patients with heart failure but no signs of congestion has been studied in only one randomised trial, which replaced diuretics with angiotensin converting enzyme inhibitors.[12]

Primary care physicians account for most diuretic prescriptions.[1] We therefore performed a double blind randomised trial among elderly patients in General Practice to assess what proportion could be successfully withdrawn from diuretic therapy.

Method Protocol
Patients aged 65 or more who had been receiving diuretics for at least six months and had no overt heart failure or hypertension were eligible for the

trial. By scanning the pharmacy registers of eight General Practices, we identified 470 patients receiving long-term diuretic therapy, of whom 268 were excluded because of a history of acute heart failure, defined as admission to hospital or prescription of intravenous diuretic therapy (27); symptoms of heart failure during the previous three months (21); manifest heart failure, defined as a heart failure score (see below) of over 4 (39); use of frusemide at dosages over 80 mg/day (26); mean of three blood pressure values (two measured at successive home visits and one obtained from the medical file) >180/100 mmHg (21); hypercalciuria, nephrotic syndrome, and glaucoma (2); use of fixed combinations of diuretics with β blockers or angiotensin converting enzyme inhibitors (25); combination therapy of β blockers, diuretics, and vasodilators for hypertension (2); use of a diuretic for which no placebo was available (40); and non-compliance during the run-in phase (1). In addition, 57 patients or their General Practitioners refused to co-operate and seven eligible patients could not be enrolled in the trial for logistic reasons.

Each General Practitioner filled out a questionnaire to assess the patient's current indications for diuretic treatment. The sample size calculation was based on the assumption that a difference of 20% between the interventions was clinically relevant and a formula was used as given by Pocock.[13] The protocol was approved by the medical ethics committee of Erasmus University/Academic Hospital Dijkzigt Rotterdam and written informed consent was obtained from all patients.

Outcomes
The primary outcome variable was successful withdrawal from diuretic therapy. Patients in the withdrawal group who were still taking blinded study medication at the end of the six month follow-up period were considered successfully withdrawn. Those patients who met one of the predefined criteria for requiring diuretic therapy within the follow-up period were considered to be unsuccessfully withdrawn. Criteria for prescription of diuretic therapy were: (a) heart failure score exceeding four points or (b) a mean of three duplicate systolic or diastolic blood pressure measurements on separate occasions of >180 mmHg or >100 mmHg respectively. Further, patients in whom diuretic therapy was restarted by their doctor for other reasons – for example, symptoms of increased shortness of breath – were considered to be unsuccessfully withdrawn. Changes in systolic and diastolic blood pressures are presented as secondary outcomes.

Baseline Assessments and Assignment
The run-in phase of four weeks included two home visits (by EPW and CvD) to collect baseline data and perform the randomisation. At the first visit all diuretic medication was handed over to the research physician and

replaced by active run-in medication of the corresponding diuretic. At the second home visit, at the end of the run-in phase, each patient was randomly assigned to placebo (the withdrawal group) or continuation of diuretic therapy (the control group), after stratification by age (65–79 and >80 years) and type of diuretic. Blocks of four sets of study medication each consisted of two placebo and two genuine packages, which were consecutively assigned to enrolled patients. Patients with frusemide dosages of 40 or 80 mg/day went through a dose halving regimen of one and two weeks, respectively, to prevent severe rebound effects. Dose halving started immediately after randomisation and was performed double blind. Randomisation lists and numbered sets of study medication were generated by the trial pharmacist of the Academic Hospital, who also produced sealed envelopes with decoding information for emergencies.

Blinding Procedure and Drug Compliance
Matching placebo was available for the five diuretics or fixed diuretic combinations most often prescribed in our region: frusemide, chlorthalidone, hydrochlorothiazide plus triamterene, epithiazide plus triamterene, and triamterene, covering 90% of all diuretic use. The similarity of genuine and placebo tablets ensured the impossibility of recognising them by colour, form or taste. The randomisation list remained in the pharmacy of the Academic Hospital in Rotterdam, separate from the trial centre in Schoonhoven. Of the sealed envelopes one copy was kept in the trial centre and another with the patient at home (for emergencies). The codes were broken either after the assessment of the last set of data, or when a diuretic prescription was needed, in which case the primary outcome of the study became actual. This blinding procedure was tested one month after randomisation by asking both the patient and the trial doctors their opinion about the content of the trial medication. Drug compliance was checked by counting tablets and asking patients about compliance at every follow-up contact and by assessment of serum diuretic concentrations (with high pressure liquid chromatography and ultraviolet fluorescence for chlorthalidone, triamterene and frusemide) at the start and the end of the study.

Follow-up
During follow-up participants were visited six times at their homes by study physicians (EPW, CvD) – 2 days, 1 and 2 weeks and 1, 3 and 6 months after randomisation. Heart failure score and blood pressure were assessed at baseline and at all follow-up visits. Heart failure symptoms were measured by means of a scoring list, including paroxysmal nocturnal dyspnoea in the preceding week (3 points); dyspnoea on exertion in the preceding week (2 points); raised jugular venous pressure (2 points; heart rate >100 beats/min (1 point); hepatojugular reflux (1 point); lower pulmonary crepitations (1 point); S3 gallop rhythm (1 point); two sided pitting ankle oedema (1 point);

and hepatomegaly (1 point). This symptom score list was validated separately.[14]

During the study duplicate blood pressure readings were taken with an Omron HEM-403C oscillometric automatic device with the patient sitting.[15] The arm with the highest blood pressure was determined at the first session and used throughout for further measurements. An electrocardiogram was recorded at baseline.

Table 2 Patients meeting one of the predefined clinical criteria requiring re-initiation of diuretic therapy.
Results are numbers of patients

Criterion	Withdrawal group (n=102)	Control group (n=100)	Risk difference (%) (95% CI)
All	50	13	36 (22–50)
Heart failure*	25	4	21 (11–31)
Hypertension*	9	5	4 (-3–11)
Subjective shortness of breath	6	0	6 (1–11)
Non-cardiac ankle oedema	4	1	3 (-1–8)
Miscellaneous clinical conditions	3	1	2 (-2–6)
Other	3	2	1 (-3–5)

*The reason for re-initiation was classified as heart failure if patients had heart failure scores >4 points and as hypertension if the mean value of three consecutive systolic or diastolic blood pressure measurements on different occasions was >180 mmHg or >100 mmHg respectively

SPECIMEN ANSWER FOR QUESTION 2

(i)   The evidence based process includes:
    1. Define an answerable question
    2. Perform literature search
             Databases e.g. Medline/Cochrane Collaboration
             Collected resources e.g. Clinical Evidence
             Review articles e.g. Bandolier
             Consider expert opinion
    3. Evaluate quality of evidence
             Consider hierarchy of evidence

(ii)
STRENGTHS
Design
- GP-based study in reputable journal
- Ethically approved and with informed consent of patients
- Double blind study
- Compliance with drug use checked objectively with blood tests

Sample
- Excluded patients with overt heart failure and/or hypertension

Outcome
- Outcome well defined
- Follow up very thorough

WEAKNESSES
Sample
- Is the assumption that a 20% difference in the two groups for significance is a valid one?
- Is the heart failure score used validated in GP use? Includes some clinical measures that seem subjective and not GP orientated (JVP, S3 gallop)

Lost Data and Bias
- How did they select the eight practices and why did 57 doctors refuse to participate? Possible introduction of bias.
- Large number of albeit well defined exclusion criteria – is this realistic in practice?
- Foreign study – is this representative of UK Practice?

(iii)

CONCLUSIONS

- About 50% of patients need to restart the diuretic for significant reasons (failure/hypertension)
- Intense follow-up is required
- Most patients seem to restart the diuretic within four weeks – perhaps the drug should be tailed off more gradually
- All patients in this study took either placebo or active treatment – the placebo effect may be significant
- The recurrence of ankle oedema may not be a problem (confidence interval crosses zero)

QUESTION 3

Mr O, a 35-year-old radiographer, presents with palpitations and anxiety. You hear an innocent systolic murmur. He asks if he ought to have an echocardiogram 'just to make sure everything is OK'.

(i) List the strengths and weaknesses of the study abstract in relation to Mr O's clinical situation.

(ii) Briefly state whether the results of this study would affect your management of Mr O.

Paper reference: McDonald *et al*; 'Opening Pandora's Box: the unpredictability of reassurance by a normal test'; BJM 1996; 313:329.

Reprinted with the kind permission of the *British Medical Journal*.

Introduction

Reassurance of patients concerned about a possible health problem is perhaps the commonest clinical transaction of all. Clinicians and textbooks generally assume that reassurance must logically follow a clear and confident statement that no disease has been found. Failure of reassurance may then be ascribed to neurosis or labelled as abnormal illness behaviour.[1] The anxiety which remains can seriously impair quality of life and result in unnecessary re-investigations, which are a burden on both the patient and the healthcare system. Despite the manifest importance of patient reassurance there has been remarkably little empirical study. We investigated this issue on the assumption that 'The scientific resolution of most problems in clinical medical management will come from analyses of events and observations that occur in non-experimental circumstances during the interaction of nature, people, technological artefacts and clinical practitioners.'[2]

Study Population and Methods

Six cardiologists in private practice and with university affiliation were each asked to recruit 10 consecutive patients who were referred to one of three laboratories (one public, two private) for the exclusion of heart disease. No cardiologist refused. Three recruited patients as requested and the remainder provided 10 patients between them. The sample of 40 patients recruited was sufficient to allow analysis in each major data category according to the principle of theoretical sampling.[3] Twenty-five patients were female and 15 male, and their average age was 32 years (range 3–74).

The symptomatic group (10 patients) presented because they were worried by symptoms, usually palpitations or chest pain or both. In the incidental group (30 patients) referral was for assessment of a systolic murmur detected during a routine examination in primary care (21 patients) or in the course of a pre-employment or insurance check (nine patients). A systolic murmur had been heard in 36 patients. Doubt had previously been raised about the heart in 13 patients – in one no fewer than four times – and echocardiography had been performed previously in six. Three patients had previously taken medication for the heart.

Data Acquisition and Analysis
Data analysed consisted of medical records, transcripts of tape recordings of the medical consultation in which the cardiologist had explained the test result, structured interviews with the cardiologists and semi-structured patient interviews.

The *cardiologist interview*, conducted by a consultant cardiologist, utilised a questionnaire developed for a previous study.[4] Data recorded included the reason for ordering the test, plans for patient management and gradings of perceived patient anxiety before and after the test. The pre-test likelihood of cardiac normality was expressed as a grading on an ordinal scale of probabilities developed by a consensus method for the earlier study,[4] in which 'probable' represented a subjective probability estimate between 0.65 and 0.89, 'almost certain' a subjective probability estimate between 0.90 and 0.99 and 'certain' a subjective probability estimate of more than 0.99. Patients were interviewed twice by a sociologist.

Patient interviews – The initial home interview was conducted as soon as possible after the medical consultation in which the test result had been explained (average 6.3 days). The follow-up home interview, conducted 9–12 months later, concentrated on subsequent progress and related medical events. One patient could not be located for the initial interview. Four patients were unavailable for follow-up; all had changed address (one had moved interstate, one overseas).

These home interviews, roughly two hours long, were structured along the lines of routine medical history taking. Thus patients were encouraged to give a free account of their perceptions and problems and leading questions were kept to a minimum to ensure that the issues discussed were those of most concern to the patient. A short checklist of direct questions, introduced as necessary at the end of the interview, was analogous to the clinical review of systems.

Analysis of transcripts – The protocol used for analysis of transcripts drew on an earlier study of patient responses.[5] Definitions of study variables and of the criteria used for their classification and grading have been reported.[6] So too have the details of the method and the results of qualitative analysis of the data.[7]

Grading quality of consultation – For the clinical consultations the important issues were what the cardiologist actually told the patient and generation of a grading of the quality of the consultation. An aggregate score was constructed as follows. A consultation was graded as 'good' if (a) explicit information about the heart was stated clearly and with confidence, (b) the patient was provided with clear and persuasive reasons for the query and referral and (c) the patient's views were elicited and discussed. The grading was 'fair' if criterion (a) was met plus either (b) or (c). In all other cases the grading was 'poor'

Patient recall and understanding – At issue in the initial patient home interview were the accuracy of the patient's recall of what the cardiologist had said, level of understanding concerning the normality of the heart, and evidence of anxiety related to doubt or misunderstanding. Patient recall of the consultation was compared with what the cardiologist had actually said according to the transcript. From the patient's own account we graded pre-test understanding as a composite index taking account of (a) understanding of the reason for the heart query and (b) understanding of the fact that serious disease was possible but unlikely. Post-test understanding was graded with respect to (a) understanding of the nature of the presenting symptoms or murmur and (b) appropriate acceptance that the heart was normal and the consequent implications for health. We graded the level of patient anxiety both before the test and after explanation of the normal result.

Observer agreement determined by comparison of the independent gradings made by a cardiologist (IMcD) and a sociologist (JD) has been presented in detail elsewhere.[6] Differences in mean observer gradings were not significant at the 5% level for any variable (Mann-Whitney U test).[8] When results for all four level grading scales were pooled there was complete agreement between observers[9] for 75.0% of gradings, minor disagreement (one grade) for 17.4% and serious disagreement (two grades) for 7.7% (Cohen's weighted κ 0.78; 95% confidence interval 0.73–0.81).[10] Agreement was therefore deemed to be satisfactory for 92.3% of gradings. Having documented the reproducibility of our application of the study protocol, the cardiologist and sociologist then graded each variable by consensus using direct quotations from the transcripts as supporting evidence. Of a total of 106 variables measured in the original study, consensus could not be reached on two, which were then eliminated from the study.

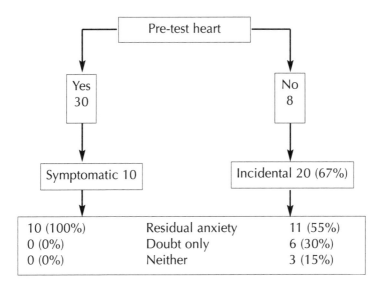

Fig 1. – *Patient's responses to test (echocardiogram) and explanation of normal result*

SPECIMEN ANSWER FOR QUESTION 3

(i)
STRENGTHS
Sample
- Age range relevant
- Clinical scenario fits, i.e. sample includes patients with normal hearts, functional murmurs and cardiac symptoms

Assessment Tool
- Made assessments of possible inter- and intra-observer bias

WEAKNESSES
Sample
- Seems small despite statistical comments
- Is this the most appropriate study design? Absence of control group is a particular problem.

Lost Data and Bias
- Private practice patients from a university setting in secondary or even tertiary care
- Consecutive selection may introduce bias (may be a particular sort of specialist session)
- 10% patients lost to follow-up
- Did the study process increase anxiety? Possible contamination of results.

Assessment Tools
- Was the system for analysing consultation quality validated? It seems basic.
- How was patient anxiety measured? Could this have been more blinded?
- A single observer used in the cardiologist interview – intra-observer error possible. This was checked – 'minor' or more significant disagreement 'in 25% of gradings'. What does this mean? Who defined the major/minor scale? Suggests inter-observer variation and reduced reliability of assessments.
- Not clear how many interviewers conducted home assessments – possible inter-observer bias. Why was more than one used?

Follow-up
- Patients seen as soon as possible after interview – but actually at average of six days. If the aim was as soon as possible why the delay?
- Follow up for 9–12 months – does anxiety settle with time? No check on this or any other factors that may have been relevant.

(ii)
This study probably has little relevance to General Practice. The success of reassurance is likely to lie within 'category (c)' listed in the method, i.e. eliciting and discussing the patient's views. The results show 100% of symptomatic (10/10) patients had residual anxiety but do not relate this to the 'quality' of the consultation. A test on its own is not helpful and that is perhaps not surprising.

Overall:
1. Study of little help to GP
2. Quality of consultation is the probable key
3. Tests applied with simple reassurance are probably unhelpful

QUESTION 4

You are writing a protocol for minor surgery in your practice. You are considering the proposal that all specimens removed should be sent for histology.
(i) List the strengths and weaknesses of the study abstract relevant to your consideration.
(ii) Explain, with justification, which points of this study you think should influence your protocol design.

Paper reference: Lowy *et al*; 'Is histological examination of tissue removed by GPs always necessary? Before and after comparison of detection rates of serious skin lesions'; BMJ 1997; 315:406.

Reprinted with the kind permission of the *British Medical Journal*.

Introduction
Since the changes to General Practitioners' contracts in 1990[1] the volume of minor surgery by General Practitioners has increased substantially.[2] Around 40% of lesions excised by General Practitioners are not referred to a pathologist.[3][4] Several researchers have reported diagnostic errors and incomplete excision of malignant lesions by General Practitioners[5-9] and have recommended mandatory pathological examination, a proposal supported by the Royal College of General Practitioners and other professional bodies.[10]

Whether this policy would benefit patients is unclear. Research has been restricted to specimens that General Practitioners have chosen to send, undoubtedly introducing a bias towards 'problematic' lesions. Nothing is known about the histological nature of lesions that General Practitioners discard. Most are clinically diagnosed as ingrown toenails, foreign bodies, skin tags, warts, ganglia, cysts and other benign lesions,[4] so it is possible that a few serious lesions are currently discarded. Although histological examination cannot harm the patient and might help, this alone does not necessarily constitute grounds for investigation, a principle that is widely accepted in other areas of clinical practice (X-ray examinations, for example, are not automatically performed after head injury[11] or ankle inversion[12] because this approach is acknowledged to result in wasteful over-investigation). Paraskevopoulos and colleagues questioned the need to examine all tissue excised during minor operations in hospital, concluding that the risks of missing an important diagnosis seemed exceptionally small for what appeared to be a considerable saving in time and money.[13]

General Practitioners probably discard about 250,000 excision specimens annually;[4] at about £18 each[3] it would cost £4.5m a year to examine them all. The Royal College of Pathologists recommends that a consultant pathologist examines 2,000–3,000 surgical specimens a year.[14] Although specimens from minor surgery are often straightforward to examine, Paraskevopoulos and colleagues suggest that 5,000 such specimens would represent a year's work for a consultant.[13] It is not known whether the benefits of examining histologically the specimens that General Practitioners discard would outweigh the cost in pathologists' time (or indeed whether any benefit would result),[15] and we examined what the impact of such a policy would be.

Method
We randomly selected 24 pathology laboratories in England.[16] Three pathologists refused to take part, one because of impending retirement and two because of concern about workload. We also randomly selected, in the catchment area of each laboratory, 8–18 General Practitioner partnerships offering minor surgery. Partnerships were excluded if they performed fewer than four excisions a month or if they had merged or split, changed the number of partners, or extended or restricted their provision of minor surgery since September 1991 (or anticipated doing so before the end of the study).

The practices agreed to obtain a histological diagnosis from their usual laboratory on all solid tissue removed by any minor surgery (including cautery and diathermy) from 1 September 1993 to 28 February 1994. Histological diagnosis, date of surgery and practice code were collected from pathology reports for all specimens sent by the practices during the intervention period and during a six month control period (1 September 1992 to 28 February 1993) before the intervention.

Two of the 21 areas were excluded because of problems with their databases. The effects of the intervention were estimated as differences in incidence; when we found evidence against a uniform intervention effect this was taken account of in stratified random-effect analyses.

Results
Of 330 partnerships in the 19 areas, 257 (response rate 78%) took part (914 General Practitioners, 1.6 million person years and 10,153 specimens). The overall referral rates increased by 29% (table 1). Although the impact on referral rates varied significantly between the areas ($\chi^2 = 162$, df = 18, P < 0.001), this appeared to be due simply to the large variation between practices, rather than to a true area effect. A random-effect analysis, in which the underlying intervention effect was considered to vary between practices, showed an average increase in referrals of 1.34 specimens per 1,000 person years (95% confidence interval 0.93–1.76).

The impact of the intervention on the detection of malignant and pre-malignant lesions was negligible (table 2), with the small falls in malignant lesions probably being the result of chance. The bulk of the increased number of referrals comprised viral warts, seborrhoeic keratoses and ingrown toenails (1,729 in the control period, 2,886 during the intervention; difference in detection rate 1.4 lesions per 1,000 person years (95% confidence interval 1.3 to 1.6 $P < 0.001$)); the increase in other benign lesions was smaller (2,409 v 2,720; 0.38 (0.21–0.56, $P < 0.001$)).

Table 1 Referral rates of tissue specimens sent by General Practitioners in intervention and control periods

Period	No. of specimens referred	Rate per 1,000 person years	Adjusted rate difference (95% CI)
Control period	4,430	5.49	11 per 1,000 person years
Intervention period	5,723	7.08	(0.93–1.76)*

* $P < 0.001$

Table 2 Malignant and pre-malignant skin lesions detected in control and intervention periods

Type of lesion	Control period	Intervention period	Detection rate difference (lesions/million person years 95% CI)
Pre-malignant lesions	91	98	9 (-25–42)
Malignant lesions:	204	188	-20 (-68–28)
Non-melanoma malignancy	188	173	-18.6 (-65–28)
Malignant melanoma	16	15	-1.2 (-15–12)
Malignant and pre-malignant lesions	295	286	-11.1 (-70–47)

SPECIMEN ANSWER FOR QUESTION 4

(i)
STRENGTHS
Design
* Very large random sample

Data Collection
* Fairly good response rate (78%)

WEAKNESSES
Design
* Was six months a suitable study period? Natural variations in number of samples may hide any intervention effect. A longer time period may even this effect out.

Lost Data
* 3/24 pathologists refused to take part – possible bias
* Why exclude partnerships with low numbers? – maybe that this is the most important group to study
* Why exclude merged/split practices or ones that had extended/ restricted services since 1991? – possible distortion of results
* 2/21 had 'problems with their database'. Why? Possible bias introduced by this 10% loss of data.

(ii)
POINTS THAT WOULD INFLUENCE PROTOCOL

* Sending all specimens increases referral rates by 29% BUT: this actually means only about two extra specimens per GP per year
* Wide confidence intervals in Table 2 make extrapolation from the results difficult – suggests the sample was too small
* Detection rates of malignancies were not influenced by the intervention
* A large proportion of the increase in samples sent for histology were warts/toenails i.e. lesions where there is no suggestion of malignancy

It would seem that sending all samples as a blanket rule is not necessary – it would increase laboratory workload with no clinical benefit.

QUESTION 5

You are interested in how parents experience difficulties when coping with acute illness in young children. Your literature search identifies the following paper, a section of which is presented.

(i)   Comment on the use of a qualitative approach for this study
(ii) Discuss the methodology as presented in this section

Paper reference: Kai J; 'Parents' difficulties and information needs in coping with acute illness in preschool children: qualitative study.'; BMJ 1996; 313:987–990.

Subjects and Methods

The methods used and the sample interviewed have been described in detail in the accompanying paper.[1] Semi-structured, one to one interviews were conducted with a purposeful sample of 32 parents living in a disadvantaged community who had at least one child under 5 years old. A further 63 parents attending three parent and toddler groups participated in focus group interviews. The interviews explored parents' experiences and difficulties coping with ill young children and were audiotaped and transcribed. Data collection and analysis used grounded theory methodology.[2] Data gathered concerning information needs were analysed using manifest content analysis.[3]

Results

The dominant theme that emerged in the analysis was of parents feeling relatively disempowered when dealing with acute illness in their children. They encountered difficulties making sense of their child's illness. Their experiences of seeking advice from professionals could leave them feeling uncertain and uninformed. The disparity between parents' beliefs and expectations about illness and treatment and professionals' behaviour further frustrated parents' attempts to understand their children's illness. These factors could act as sources of dissatisfaction and sometimes disharmony in the relationship between parent and doctor.

'It's just a virus' – assessment and information sharing by doctors

Parents were generally confident about recognising whether their child was becoming ill. They used combinations of behavioural and symptomatic clues assessed against any deviation from what was normal for their particular child. There was far more uncertainty about deciding what was wrong and if a problem was significant or serious. Parents drew on family, friends, or the local pharmacy for guidance but usually consulted, or were advised to consult, their doctor when an illness was causing them concern.

Respondents were curious to know how doctors evaluated an ill child. They felt excluded from the apparent mystique of the professional's assessment. The commonest example was seeking advice about a child's cough when they feared infection 'on the chest' because the child's chest sounded, and even felt 'rattley.' However, the doctor would pronounce the lungs 'clear' on examination despite apparent evidence to the contrary. Parents would then find it difficult to question the doctor's authority and were left feeling silly for worrying or still perplexed by the problem. Parents also often wondered how doctors determined the severity of illness in babies (Box 1).

Box 1 – The mystique of the doctor's assessment

'When the little one's sounding raspy and wheezy…the doctor sort of puts the stethoscope on and says, 'Well, it sounds clear,' but I mean you know yourself there's something wrong' (Parent 15)

'She was bringing back her bottles and I thought she was really sick…He came and took one look and said she was OK, but how did he know?' (Parent 24)

SPECIMEN ANSWER FOR QUESTION 5

(i) **Use of Qualitative Approach**
- Appropriate to use qualitative approach
- Attempts to describe and understand the individual, and collective experiences of people
- Attempt at obtaining a 'rich description' of the phenomenon under investigation

(ii) **STRENGTHS**
- Good description of context – disadvantaged inner city community
- Purposive sampling performed. This approach aims to reflect the diversity within a given population rather than statistical generalisability.
- All interviews audiotaped and transcribed
- Focus group interviews performed on a larger population. This is an attempt to triangulate data to provide increased validity and generalisability.
- Data collection and analysis using grounded theory approach. This methodology produces categories that are derived from the data rather than the questions on the interview schedule or focus group topic guide. These concepts are those expressed by the respondents, reflecting how they perceive the phenomenon rather than the researcher.
- Categories supported by relevant direct quotations from parents

WEAKNESSES
- Possible researcher bias during the interviewing, transcription and data analysis. No quality checks performed.
- No statement about respondent validation. This involves returning the research findings to the original respondents to check that the researcher has correctly reflected their perceptions. (This was actually done by the author but is described only in the earlier quoted paper.)

QUESTION 6

A six partner seaside General Practice reviews its prescribing costs. The following data was obtained:

	Cost per own patient (£)	Cost per temporary resident (TR) (£)
GIT drugs	1.56	0.30
Cardiovascular drugs	1.58	0.25
Respiratory drugs	1.01	0.21
CNS drugs	1.02	0.18
Anti-infectives	0.54	1.59
Endocrine drugs	0.62	0.14
Joint disease drugs	0.83	0.20
Skin preparations	0.41	0.78
Vaccines	0.03	0.04
Dressings	0.23	0.17

The comparative costs of the various drugs used by temporary residents as opposed to the practice's own patients.

Comment on the presented data, giving possible explanations for your observations.

SPECIMEN ANSWER FOR QUESTION 6

* Lowered costs per patient noted for TR in all areas except anti-infectives, skin preparations and vaccines, with only slight reduction in dressings.
* It is not stated if the average cost is over the whole year or just one quarter. Possibly only over busy summer quarter when there is an influx of seaside visitors.

Factors in patients

a) Increased TR costs

Increased infections, especially minor, e.g. URTI. In considering increased vaccines and only slightly reduced dressings costs, possibility of increased wound infections, receiving tetanus booster and dressings. Increase in minor skin disorders, especially sunburn or skin irritations.

b) Reduced TR costs

Little long-term prescribing for major prescribing areas, especially CNS. Possibly reflects younger population of visitors and that they obtained long-term medications from their own GP before visiting area.

Factors in Doctors

a) Possibly little patient education (altering patients' health beliefs and health-seeking behaviour) for minor infections and skin irritations.

b) 'Symptom' prescribing for minor problems, related to temporary residents' expectations, volume of workload, patients' psychosocial factors and whether seen at surgery or at home visit.

QUESTION 7

Comment on the presented data, giving possible explanations for your observations.

GP DIRECT ACCESS PHYSIOTHERAPY SERVICE	
Number of referrals received	176
Total number of patients seen	157
Number Failed 1st appointment	31
Unable to attend	47
Did not attend	16

Signed.

Head of Physiotherapy
Community Physiotherapy Service

SPECIMEN ANSWER FOR QUESTION 7

- The presented data and the table are unclear:

a) 'Failed 1st appointment' and 'did not attend' amalgamated to produce – 'Unable to Attend' or are all three categories separate?
b) How are the categories 'failed 1st appointment', 'unable to attend' and 'did not attend' distinguished?
c) Whatever combination is considered, they do not reflect the difference between 'Number of Referrals Received' and 'Total Number of Patients seen'

- Approximately 11% of referrals made are not seen. This does not seem to be unreasonable, but there are wasted appointments.
- Failure to attend first appointment may be due to several factors e.g.
  - long waiting list, with resolution of problem or seeking of alternative
  - private referral, inconvenient time or date
- Further information on the categories is essential before meaningful conclusions can be made

QUESTION 8

Catheter Care – Practice Protocol

Long Term Catheters are associated with a number of complications – blockage, bypassing, stone formation and periurethral abscesses. These may be minimised by correct care.

1. Avoid kinking of drainage tube.
2. Avoid constipation – regular laxatives will help.
3. Maintain a high fluid intake.
4. Arrange plain abdominal X-ray if bladder stone is suspected – refer if confirmed.
5. Ascorbic acid 1 g tds acidifies urine and may decrease stone formation.
6. Bendrofluazide 5 mg nocte will decrease phosphate encrustation.
7. Bladder washouts do little to help and should be avoided.
8. If bypassing is a problem ensure catheter is not blocked, try Probanthine 15 mg tds. If problem persists a suprapubic catheter may be the answer – refer for this.
9. Periurethral abscesses require antibiotics and possibly admission and drainage if the patient is ill.

You are presented with this protocol. List recommendations for improving the protocol, giving your reasons.

SPECIMEN ANSWER FOR QUESTION 8

Recommendations for improvements

Purpose and scope
* Clear description of patient group to whom it will apply and the healthcare providers who will be applying it e.g. age and sex range
* Identification of who is responsible for the development of the protocol e.g. primary or secondary care/medical or nursing staff

Clinical flexibility
* Specific information about situations in which clinical exceptions might be made on applying the protocol e.g. spinal injuries or after stroke

Validity
* Specific description of methods used to collect the evidence on which the recommendations in the protocol are based
* Adequate supporting references
* Are they evidence-based?
* Are they mere anecdote?
* Comparison with other guidelines, protocols or expert reviews

Multidisciplinary process
* Clear description of who participated in the development of the protocol
* Any potential biases should be noted e.g. commercial sponsorship

Likely cost and benefits
* Discussion of both financial and patient cost-benefit outcomes for the recommendations

Clarity
* Need for clear and unambiguous presentation

Clinical audit
* Should state specific criteria for monitoring compliance of protocol

Review and updating
- Specific date for reviewing or updating stated
- Description of who will be responsible and how it will be reviewed or updated

QUESTION 9

Use of dipstick haematuria in the detection of carcinoma of the bladder

A practice screens 459 men between 60 and 80 years with dipstick for haematuria, referring any positive results for urological investigation. The results obtained are:

		DISEASE STATUS	
		Carcinoma of bladder – Present	No carcinoma of bladder detected
Dipstick haematuria	Positive	4	8
	Negative	1	446

What is the sensitivity and specificity and positive predictive value of this test?

SPECIMEN ANSWER FOR QUESTION 9

Sensitivity: possibility of a positive test in people with disease

$$: \quad \frac{\text{Number of true positives}}{\text{Number of true positives + number of false negatives}}$$

$$: \quad \frac{4}{4+1} \quad = 80\%$$

Specificity: probability of a negative test in people without the disease

$$: \quad \frac{\text{Number of true negatives}}{\text{Number of false positives + number of true negatives}}$$

$$: \quad \frac{446}{8+446} \quad = 98\%$$

Positive predictive: probability of the person having the disease when the test is value positive

$$: \quad \frac{\text{Number of true positives}}{\text{Number of true positives + number of false positives}}$$

$$: \quad \frac{4}{4+8} \quad = 33\%$$

This is low since the prevalence of the condition is low.

QUESTION 10

PRACTICE ANNUAL REPORT

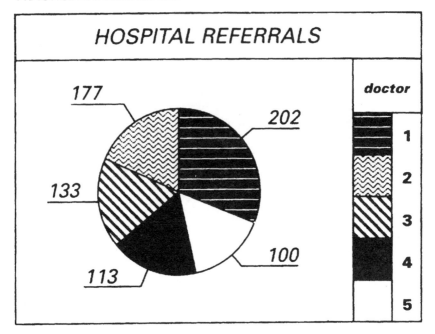

1. Comment on the above data.

2. What are the possible causes of variation in hospital referrals made by each doctor?

SPECIMEN ANSWER FOR QUESTION 10

1.
- The candidate is expected to demonstrate the ability to extract information from a pie chart.
- Doctor 1 has 202 hospital referrals, over twice that of doctor 5 (100) and also significantly more than any other doctor in the practice. Doctor 2 is the next highest referrer with 177.
- Appreciation of limitation of gross figures, without further information e.g. list size, part/full time partners, etc.
- Uncertainty of what it relates to e.g. is it in-patient, which specialty and to which hospitals?

2.
- Appreciation of wide variety of hospital referrals between individual doctors and that many factors involved.
- Appreciation of difficulties when no further breakdown of information e.g. whether referred to in-patients or out-patients and which individual specialties. Also whether includes patient self-referrals e.g. to casualty departments.
- Appreciation of various factors involved:

   a) **Patients** – the doctor may look after a particular group of patients with problems requiring referral e.g. elderly in nursing homes.

   b) **GP** – special interest e.g. increased referrals for certain specialist investigation. Poorer confidence when dealing with problems in a General Practice setting. Different personal list sizes, including whether trainer and trainee referrals added to responsible partner's figures. Availability e.g. part-time partners or holidays and sick/maternity leave during the study period.

APPROACH TO CURRENT AWARENESS TYPE QUESTIONS

Current awareness questions examine candidates' knowledge of the literature in relation to current practice. Candidates are expected to be familiar with items in the medical literature which have influenced current thinking and relevant issues in General Practice.

This type of question tests candidates' ability to:
- Give an account of their current state of knowledge of a major topic relevant to General Practice
- Support this account with reference to background literature
- Critically appraise the evidence to decide whether it has clinical relevance to General Practice
- Identify and discuss areas of controversy with a logical argument

The following are examples of typical questions which have appeared in the examination:

- Summarise current thinking on antidepressant medication.
- Evaluate the place of self-monitoring in asthma.
- What is the evidence for the value of counsellors in General Practice?

How Questions are Chosen
Questions will have been chosen because they are about issues which are important and very relevant to General Practice. It is very likely that there will be recent published scientific evidence relating to the topic on which clinical and practice management can be based. Candidates should remember, however, that many older studies also have considerable influence.

A list of topics of current awareness-type questions which have appeared in recent examinations is shown in the table overleaf.

Hot Topics questions appearing in Paper 1 in the 2000 and 2001 exams

May 2000	Diabetes mellitus (glycaemic control, self monitoring & blood pressure control) Anti-coagulation monitoring Rationing	**May 2001**	Heart failure Revalidation Practice Web site Refugees Opiate abuse
October 2000	Hypertension Osteoporosis Atrial fibrillation Treatment of Alzheimer's disease Polycystic ovary syndrome Benign prostatic hypertrophy	**October 2001**	Otitis media Rheumatoid arthritis Frozen shoulder Back pain Smoking cessation

A candidate examining this list will recognise that it contains topics which are always going to be relevant such as diabetes, hypertension and alcohol abuse. Mixed with these are subjects which are more topical and about which there have been many recent papers. There may have been advances in treatment, such as in heart failure or the use of lipid-lowering drugs, or there may have been controversy, such as in screening for prostate cancer or prescribing third generation combined oral contraceptives. It should not therefore be too difficult for candidates to identify likely questions. Potential questions are tested on a large number of examiners before being adopted, so it is unlikely that obscure topics will pass through.

How to Answer Questions

Candidates often express concern about answering current awareness questions. This concern centres on uncertainty about how to display knowledge of the medical literature and in particular on the need to quote references. When examiners design a question they also produce a model answer based on published literature. A candidate who is able to identify the main points in the answer will obtain a good mark. The use of relevant references will move the mark higher, particularly if some appraisal of these takes place. The following example outlines a question and its model answer:

EXAMPLE QUESTION 1

Discuss the quality of care of patients with epilepsy in General Practice. What strategies have been suggested for improvement?

Answer

- Epilepsy is a common chronic illness (point prevalence 0.4–1.0%). Up to 90% are not under hospital supervision yet epilepsy has been left out of the chronic disease management payments.
- Problems that have been identified with quality of care include inaccurate diagnoses, lack of systematic follow-up, under treatment, polypharmacy, poor compliance, failure in GP–patient communication and a low level of recording detail in notes.
- The following barriers have been identified:
  - The organisation of care including a lack of disease registers in practices and lack of support from hospitals where patients are often seen by non-neurologists.
  - The General Practitioner who often lacks knowledge and motivation and may worry about time and the cost of care.
  - The patient who may have a low motivation to seek help often due to the stigma of epilepsy. He may also have poor knowledge about his condition and be further complicated by co-existing mental or physical illness.
- Two major nationwide initiatives have been established to improve care:
  - The epilepsy task force, a multidisciplinary group, which evolved from the panel of experts who produced the 'epilepsy needs document'. Its broad aims include a public awareness campaign, improved primary and secondary care provision, research and audit to improve services in primary care and the introduction of guidelines for management.(Brown *et al* 1993.)
  - A liaison nurse programme between a hospital specialist epilepsy clinic and General Practice. (Wellcome foundation 1993.)

All of the material used in this answer was contained in a review article in the British Journal of General Practice just over 12 months before the exam (Thapar 1996). Several other articles were also published in that period and some marks would be obtained by identifying the points outlined in the model answer. Remembering where you had read about them would be less important. The information above cannot be found in textbooks so it could only have been acquired by reading recent papers.

The outline represents a perfect answer. In the short time available in the examination it is unlikely that anyone could reproduce it. It may be helpful therefore to look at what standard of answer would give a high score in terms of marks, an average score and a low score.

Range of answers and their marks

High mark: Candidates would demonstrate a wide knowledge touching at least in brief on most aspects of the model answer. It would be very clear that they had read Thapar's review article and would probably quote other references as well.

Average mark: About half the points would be identified either evenly spread through most areas of the answer or covering one or two areas in depth (usually problems identified and barriers to care) and missing others. The use of references would usually be superficial.

Low mark: One or two areas would be touched upon but only superficially and probably by chance. Many candidates would write about the clinical management of epilepsy (investigations, drugs, monitoring, etc.). Any references would be irrelevant.

In some questions being able to quote references is more important. These references will usually relate to large, much publicised trials, review articles or campaigns. The example below is such a question. It also shows a variation from the traditional style of question. Here clinical scenarios are presented.

EXAMPLE QUESTION 2

Discuss any published evidence which might influence you to attempt blood pressure after serial management is shown:

1. A man of 58 years. He has type 2 diabetes mellitus. Blood pressure 150/85.
2. A man of 40 years. His 45-year-old brother has angina. His father died of a myocardial infarction aged 50 years. Blood pressure 145/92.
3. A woman of 70 years with no cardiovascular risk factors or adverse clinical findings. Blood pressure is persistently elevated at 175/95.

Answer

In all three cases there are grounds for recommending treatment because:

- The target blood pressure for diabetic patients is 140/80 from the BHS guidelines.
- The benefits are also seen in elderly people (Amery *et al* 1985, SHEP Co-operative research group 1991, Medical Research Council Working Party 1992).
- The British Hypertension Society would recommend treatment.

Further marks could be obtained in this question by pointing out that trials have used mainly diuretics and b-blockers. However, the evidence is for the actual reduction in blood pressure rather than the methods and drugs used. Treatment should also be considered depending on a patient's other cardiovascular risk factors. Also, candidates would be expected to discuss the value of non-pharmacological methods of treatment and consider the importance of other risk factors.

The question looks for evidence in favour of treating mild hypertension. The scenarios involve a person with target organ damage, a person with a strong cardiovascular risk factor and an elderly person. The most important publication on this subject are the British Hypertension Society Guidelines (BMJ 1999;319:630) and all candidates would be expected to show evidence of having read this.

It may be that you will find a question for which it will be difficult to find references from your recent reading of the journals which are relevant to the questions being asked. It is important to resist quoting articles which are related but not directly relevant. Rather, write an answer stating what you know about the subject being questioned. An example of a question which might cause this sort of difficulty is shown below.

EXAMPLE QUESTION 3

Discuss the benefits of hormone replacement therapy for the prevention of:
a)   cardiovascular disease   b) osteoporosis.

Answer

a)   Cardiovascular disease:
- Oestrogen has been shown to reduce LDL cholesterol and probably raises HDL cholesterol
- The HERS study showed that HRT can reduce the rate of cardiovascular events (but there was an increase in events in the first year of the trial)
- It is not possible to recommend HRT to women with established IHD at an older age
- Further randomised controlled trials are underway to clarify the association of HRT and IHD

b)   Osteoporosis:
- Oestrogen decreases the rate of absorption of trabecular bone principally by inhibition of osteoclastic activity
- Numerous prospective placebo-controlled studies show that oestrogens reduce the long term risk of fracture of the hips (by about 30%), wrist and spine (by about 50%)
- To maximise skeletal benefits treatment should be started at the time of the menopause because this is the time of accelerated bone loss

---

> - Bone loss may be arrested at any age but bone loss will not be restored
> - To gain maximum benefit HRT should be taken for at least five years and longer if there has been a premature menopause
> - 10 years after stopping HRT the bone density and fracture risk are similar to women who have never taken HRT

A high scoring candidate would identify seven or more of these points and a poor scoring candidate less than three. Evidence of reading and the insertion of more detail would also influence the final mark.

For many of these current awareness questions there may well be other important issues which are not the sort of issues which could be supported by evidence. So, for instance, in the care of a patient after a myocardial infarction, the General Practitioner is important for providing continuity of care for both the patient and the family, for their skills as a communicator and for their insight into the social and psychological processes which might affect the outcome. These and other similar attributes of a General Practitioner and their interaction with patients are examined elsewhere in the written papers. It is important to distinguish questions requiring evidence from those which do not in order to avoid wasted effort, for in a current awareness question discussion of such issues will not attract marks. Examination development may well result in more integration of questions and candidates will need to remain alert for possible subtle changes. The advice to 'read the question carefully' holds good even at this level.

With just over 15 minutes to answer a question it is not advisable to attempt to produce essay answers. By using an expanded note form a lot of information can be put down on paper. Also this makes it easier for examiners to mark. However if abbreviations are used it is important to make sure that they are used commonly enough for the examiner to know what they mean.

How to Prepare for the Examination

Critical reading should be a lifelong activity which is a part of our continuing professional development. However, those who feel the need to make some special preparation for the examination should concentrate on the British Medical Journal and the British Journal of General Practice. Certainly the preceding two years' issues should be worked through. The title of every article should be read and, where it has relevance for General Practice, candidates should at least continue and read the summary. Interest or the fact that the article is contributing to the body of knowledge on a 'hot topic' should inspire candidates to read further.

The topics in Table 1 could form a starting point for anyone assembling a list of 'hot topics'. It is worth gathering together papers under topic headings and keeping them in a file. Many trainers may already have done this, so all that is required is to add recent information and identify any new topics which seem important. Particularly important are editorials, review articles and many of the Occasional Papers of the Royal College of General Practitioners. These are useful for building up a wider picture of published work. In order to build up the full picture of a particular subject it may be necessary to do a library search or use Medline or the Internet. Groups of candidates meeting together to share out information gathering and discuss topics saves time and is a very useful exercise.

Candidates often worry about current awareness questions more than they do about other parts of the examination. They are only about keeping up-to-date, something which all of us should surely do. If there is a topic about which you think you know little, remember that it only forms a small proportion of the overall examination in terms of marks so there is no need to panic. Write down what you know. You are bound to score some marks.

References

Amery A, Birkenhager W, Brixo P. *et al* (1985) Mortality and morbidity results from the European Working Party in the Elderly Trial. *Lancet,* 1, 1349–1354.

Brown S, Bretts T, Chadwick D, *et al* (1993) An epilepsy needs document. *Seizure,* 2, 91–103.

Collins R, Peto R, MacMahon S, *et al* (1990) Blood pressure, stroke and coronary heart disease. Part 2. Short-term reductions in blood pressure: overview of randomised drug trials in their epidemiological context. *Lancet,* 335, 827–38.

Medical Research Council Working Party (1992) MRC trial of treatment of hypertension in older adults, principal results. *British Medical Journal*, 304, 405–12.

Sever P, Beevers G, Bulpitt C, et al (1993) Management guidelines in essential hypertension: Report of the second working party of the British Hypertension Society. *British Medical Journal*, 306, 983–7.

SHEP Co-operative Research Group (1991) Prevention of stroke by anti-hypertensive drug treatment in older persons with isolated systolic hypertension. *Journal of the American Medical Association*, 265, 3255–64.

Thapar AK (1996) Care of patients with epilepsy in the community: will new initiatives address old problems? *British Journal of General Practice*, 46, 37– 42.

Wellcome Foundation (1993) Epilepsy liaison nurse programme: a management protocol for epilepsy in general practice. Crewe, Wellcome Foundation.

Whitehead M, Godfree V, (1992) Hormone replacement therapy – your questions answered. Churchill Livingstone.

APPROACH TO PROBLEM SOLVING TYPE QUESTIONS

Paper 1 has questions which test candidates' ability to integrate and apply theoretical knowledge and professional values to practical problems encountered in an NHS setting.

There will usually be a number of clinical patient-focused questions and a number of practice-focused questions and also questions on wider issues.

The Area Covered

The candidate is expected to appreciate the whole range of problems that the average General Practitioner could expect to come across in their practice – clinical, ethical, administrative or concerning self-awareness and development.

What the Examiners are Looking For

Questions may present a problem which you have never experienced before, but the examiners are looking for the principles of problem solving which are no different to those used every day, and expect the candidate to understand the key issues that are presented. These key issues are known as constructs. A construct is a theme, a strand, a dimension, one of a number of 'nubs' the question may have.

Examples of constructs:

- Clinical competence
- Consultation and communication skills
- Awareness of patient's hidden agenda
- Recognition of patient's point of view
- Ability to predict future developments
- Cost effectiveness
- Follow-up arrangements
- Insight into family, social, occupational, environmental & cultural influences on outcome
- Preventive interventions and promotion of good health
- Financial and business acumen
- Awareness of ethical considerations
- Involvement of other team members and appropriate use of resources
- Awareness of doctor's own feelings/motivation
- Clinical safety
- 'Caritas' - sense of genuine caring or empathy
- Logical and systematic approach

Each candidate is provided with a combined question and answer booklet, and each page goes to a different examiner so it is important to not to refer to things that have been written in answer to a previous question. The examiners mark the paper by reference to how the candidate performs in the main constructs. The examiners have a marking schedule which considers five constructs per question, and these constructs are chosen to be as separate from each other as possible, so that a candidate may do well in one independently of their performance in another. Overlapping themes would unfairly penalise a candidate twice if the concept was missed.

The candidate's performance relating to each construct is graded from 0 to 5:

0	**Non existent**	No mention is made at all of the particular construct and it appears the candidate did not seem to consider it.
1	**Bad**	The candidate appears to acknowledge the construct's existence by implication or in passing but does not develop it to any degree. Its meaning may have been misunderstood, its significance not perceived or responses to it may be inappropriate.
2	**Mediocre**	The construct is explicitly mentioned but there is little evidence that it is really understood. Discussion may be sketchy or jargon-ridden. Examples may be too few or too non-specific to display an acceptable level of understanding.
3	**Satisfactory**	The candidate satisfies the examiner that the essentials of the construct are adequately understood, though without particular flair.
4	**Good**	The candidate clearly demonstrates a better grasp of the construct than most. There is good detail and description, though a few relatively minor points may be omitted.
5	**Excellent**	The candidate shows a superior coverage of the construct both in principle and in detail.

The actual constructs that the examiners use in the marking brief describe what a good candidate would be expected to do on a good day, recognising the time constraints of the surgery. It is thus important to think widely because if one construct is missed it is only possible to obtain 80% of the marks. To gain a high mark it is important to be aware of the breadth **and** the depth of each construct. The final mark will take the form of a pass, fail or merit for the best 25% or so of candidates.

How to Maximise Your Marks and How to Approach the Question

- Think yourself into the situation. Many of the questions are based on real experiences that the examiners have been through. What are the problems in the described situation? Do not forget the feelings that you may have when faced with the situation (self-awareness). It is important to think widely and divergently, and also to think how you would approach the situation on an ideal day if you had adequate time and resources.
- Think of the key themes that this question is beginning to highlight – these are the constructs.
- Write short notes on each of the constructs, expanding as much as possible so that the examiner can appreciate how much (or how little!) you know about this area. It is important to remember that the examiner is looking to see whether you actually understand what the construct is about rather than just regurgitating bland terms e.g. ideas, concerns and expectations. Many people ask: How much should I write? The secret is to try and get as much information down as you can in the allotted time per question, which is 15 minutes.
- Remember – keep a close eye on the time. Answering the questions within the time constraints is an important skill. Legible and concise note form is the preferred method.
- Don't panic!

When answering these types of questions, it is advisable to:

- Read each question carefully and answer it as it is asked
- Think in a wide-ranging way (but realistically) about how a competent and sensitive GP would deal with each scenario
- Avoid jargon, clichés and over-generalisation
- Include illustrative details, explanations and relevant examples

Example

Your Practice Manager has received a letter of complaint from a patient who has recently had a cervical smear performed by one of your male partners. The patient states that she found the procedure very embarrassing and that she felt that a chaperone should have been present.

Discuss the implications of this letter.

A good candidate will be expected to cover the following constructs:

Medico-legal   Appreciation of the need for a chaperone, respect for patient's privacy and confidentiality.

Practice organisation Review and establishment of practice policy, method of dealing with complaints.

Problem solving   Method of reply, considering the consequences of each proposed intervention.

Self-awareness   Annoyance at patient or partner. Understanding own vulnerability and concern for the future.

Duties to a colleague Empathy and support to colleague. Colleague experiencing difficulties.

PRACTICE QUESTIONS

Write your answers in the space provided. Your answers should be brief and may take the form of lists rather than lengthy descriptions. The answers are given after each question.

QUESTION 1

Gemma Smith, aged 15 years, attends accompanied by her mother. She complains of a vaginal discharge. Her mother stays in the consulting room while you examine Gemma with the practice nurse as chaperone in a separate room. She tells you that she had sexual intercourse a week ago but asks you not to tell her mother.

Outline your management.

ANSWER 1

The good candidate would be expected to consider the following:

Ethics	Gemma's autonomy and right to confidentiality, recognise that she is a minor, duty to Gemma and also her mother.
Communication	Talking to Gemma (eliciting her concerns and teenager communication difficulties), what to tell her mother, encourage her to discuss the situation with mother and family. Consideration of a practice policy for chaperones.
Clinical management	Vaginal discharge, contraception, STD, consider possibility of pregnancy, ?refer.
Prevention	Contraception, reducing risks STD/HIV, other lifestyle advice.
Practice organisation	Follow-up, consider health care and sexual health needs of teenagers. Methods of making surgery more teenager-friendly.

QUESTION 2

Brian Oatley is a 58-year-old carpenter and a heavy smoker. He has come for the result of a recent day case bronchoscopy, which revealed a bronchial carcinoma. He has not been told of the findings.

How would you handle this situation?

ANSWER 2

A good candidate would be expected to consider the following:

Communication
Establish rapport/empathy, check patient's understanding, plan hierarchy of giving information and check understanding at each stage, deal with denial/strong emotions.

Practice organisation
Make time for doctor and patient. Consider presence of spouse/friend/nurse. Use of a double appointment for this consultation.

Ethics
Patient autonomy – right to know the diagnosis but balance with right not to know information if patient does not wish. Offer patient the opportunity to say first whether he wants all the information.

Patient Centredness
Negotiation of management plan.

Clinical Management
Immediate – management of haemoptysis/other symptoms.
Long-term – referral options (two-week cancer referral), own knowledge of realistic treatment options before consultation.
Involvement of other practice team members (other partners, district nurses, Macmillan nurses etc).

Self-awareness
Feelings towards patient, feelings towards hospital. Coping with possible strong patient's reaction, readiness to see next patient.

QUESTION 3

You are on call for your practice and at 11 pm you are telephoned by Tracey Tyler. Her 5-month-old son, Billy, has been passing bright red blood in his stools for the past 24 hours.
She says he is well in himself.

What issues does this consultation raise?

ANSWER 3

A good candidate would be expected to consider the following:

Clinical management Assess medical needs, consider visit, advice over telephone.

Practice organisation Logistics of night visit, use of out of hours services, night visit fee.
Review of practice visiting policy to encourage visit requests in the mornings.

Communication Establish mother's concerns and health beliefs, clear information gathering and advice over telephone.
Pros and cons of telephone consultations.

**Altering help-
seeking behaviour** Consider principles.

Self-awareness Anger at time, minor complaint.

QUESTION 4

You are called out of surgery by Barry Tallman, who is a 67-year-old retired chef. He has a four hour history of central chest pain. He looks well and on examination he has a BP of 130/80 and a regular pulse of 98 beats per minute. You diagnose that he has a probable myocardial infarction.

How do you decide to manage him?

ANSWER 4

A good candidate would be expected to consider the following:

Clinical management   Establish diagnosis, consider use of thrombolysis (e.g. in rural setting) give immediate dose of aspirin and GTN, consider use of ECG, referral strategies.

Evidence-based approach   Knowledge of studies of home versus hospital care, knowledge of use of aspirin and thrombolysis.

Patient centredness   Patient choice/preference, patient's concerns and health beliefs.

Psychosocial awareness   Aware of psychosocial factors e.g. living alone, adverse social circumstances.

Self-awareness   Confidence/competence in dealing with the problem, ease of follow-up.

Practice organisation   Procedure for urgent visits when on-call. May have been more appropriate to call for an emergency ambulance instead of visiting the patient at home.

QUESTION 5

Carol Hanson, a 42-year-old part-time secretary, enters your surgery and bursts into tears. She states that she has just discovered that her accountant husband has been having an affair with a junior colleague.

What would you hope to achieve by the end of this consultation?

ANSWER 5

A good candidate would be expected to consider the following:

Communication   Establish rapport, negotiation of options, focus on the patient's ideas and concerns.

Clinical management Exclude depression, arrangements for follow-up.

Psychosocial support Self and friends, voluntary and statutory.

'Caritas'   Empathy and caring.

Practice organisation Time constraints during a busy surgery, arrangements for follow-up.

QUESTION 6

Jim Connoll is a 44-year-old electrician and presents with a 10 day history of low back pain, which is not settling despite rest. He would like you to refer him to an osteopath.

How would you respond?

ANSWER 6

A good candidate would be expected to consider the following:

Communication	Establish patient's ideas, concerns and health beliefs about low back pain and osteopathy, hidden agenda?
Ethics	Respect patient's autonomy about choice of alternative practitioner.
Clinical management	Management of low back pain, exclusion of serious illness, role of clinical examination.
Evidence-based approach	Guidelines on low back pain, research on benefits of osteopath versus physiotherapy.
Self-awareness	Personal views and tolerance on role of complementary medicine.

QUESTION 7

You are called into reception by your receptionist. Darren, a known drug addict, is shouting and demanding to be seen immediately.

How do you manage this situation?

ANSWER 7

A good candidate would be expected to consider the following:

Communication   Dealing with angry patients.

Practice organisation Emergency appointments, balance of priorities with other patients, reception staff training.

Teamwork   Important to have unified response, especially after traumatic event.

Clinical management Management of presenting complaint, including drug addiction.

Self-awareness   Annoyance at patient, and how it affects management of current patients and following patients.

QUESTION 8

At the end of surgery you are visited by a pharmaceutical company representative who asks if you would like to attend an all-expenses paid scientific meeting in Rome. The subject area is one which interests you.

What issues does this invitation raise?

ANSWER 8

A good candidate would be expected to consider the following:

Ethical	GMC rules on acceptance of hospitality, feeling of obligation to the representative in the future, alteration in prescribing pattern, relationship with representative in the future.
Professional Education/Self-development	Assessment of educational event, assessment of own learning needs.
Practice organisation	Time, locum cover, incidental expenses.
Problem solving	Consider cost versus benefits in attending meeting.
Self-awareness	Balancing ethical considerations against cheap method of obtaining PGEA, affect of decision on relationship with representative in the future, relationship with other colleagues in practice.

QUESTION 9

Following a clinical governance meeting in your practice, you produce a list of proposed practice audits.

How do you decide which one to proceed with?

ANSWER 9

A good candidate would be expected to consider the following:

Practice organisation Resource implications, costs versus benefits to the practice, organisational difficulties, methods and practicalities for re-auditing.

Problem solving Prioritise, relevance, feasibility, cost versus benefit considerations.

Personal and professional growth Addressing learning needs, personal commitment or enjoyment of the subject.

Teamwork Involving other members of the primary health care team and developing working relationships.

Wider NHS context Response to local health needs, National Service Framework targets, requirement for chronic disease management payments.

QUESTION 10

Your Practice Manager informs you of the need to purchase a new autoclave, costing £2000, since the old one is beyond repair.

What factors would you expect to take into account in the decision to replace it?

ANSWER 10

A good candidate would be expected to consider the following:

Problem solving   Requirement of autoclave in the future, possible further uses of autoclave, workload considerations.

Practice organisation   Delegation for maintenance, training issues.

Financial and business   Planning method of purchase/lease/hire, service contract.

Teamwork   Involve all concerned, respecting autonomy of main users e.g. practice nurse decision.

Self-awareness   Reluctance to spend large sums of money, conflicting priorities, feeling of anger or blame.

QUESTION 11

Your attached district nurse would like to introduce an evidence and research-based approach to the management of leg ulcers in your patients.

Discuss the implications of this approach.

ANSWER 11

A good candidate would be expected to consider the following:

Respect for fellow professionals Consider autonomy, training and responsibilities.

Practice organisation Protocol and referral pathways development, audit possible?

Communication Need to have common understanding of what is meant by evidence and research-based approach, hidden agenda of district nurse?

Teamwork Opportunity to work together jointly, other community staff involved or only practice nurse?

Self-awareness Lack of knowledge of the proposed approach, feelings about change and delegation of duties to nursing colleagues.

QUESTION 12

Pat, your practice nurse, is due to retire in four months' time. The partnership decides to draw up a new job description.

How would you decide what to include in the job description?

ANSWER 12

A good candidate would be expected to consider the following:

Practice organisation Hours, pay and conditions, who to report to, qualifications required.

Problem solving Logical approach considering present needs, future needs, skills mix required.

Team working Practice dynamics and type of personality required to work in existing primary health care team.

Primary care development Extended role of the practice nurse and Nurse Practitioners.

Role of professional colleague Delegation versus autonomy, health professional.

APPROACH TO MULTIPLE CHOICE AND COMPUTER-MARKED QUESTIONS

Multiple choice type questions form the basis for Paper 2 which is designed to test the extent of candidates' knowledge about General Practice, including both established and recent knowledge, and also the deeper understanding and application of that knowledge.

Questions in Paper 2 are developed by a group of examiners and are derived from reference sources, including review articles and original papers in journals readily available to all General Practitioners – this includes the *British Medical Journal*, *The British Journal of General Practice*, *Clinical Evidence* and *Drug and Therapeutics Bulletin*.

You should expect questions on a broad range of relevant General Practice key areas

- Core knowledge
- Emerging knowledge (mainly published in 18/12 before exam)
- Application of knowledge
- Critical Appraisal – including knowledge of statistics and research methodology sufficient to evaluate published papers

Format of Paper 2

The paper contains a number of different format questions. For example, it will consist of extended matching items, single best answers, multiple best answers and tables or written material to appraise either in any of these formats or by selecting the most appropriate word from a menu of choices reflecting the most accurate critique.

The number of standard true/false items has been steadily reduced over recent years and, in May 2002, the format was abolished and the number of items reduced. The college has also stated that it intends to increase the number of images (including fundi, skins, ECGs etc) used in this paper in the future.

EXAMPLE QUESTIONS

SINGLE BEST ANSWER (SBA) QUESTIONS
These consist of a statement or stem followed by a variable number of items, only one of which is correct.

Example of SBA Question

In the management of croup in a 2-year-old child, which single best treatment has been shown in a randomised-controlled trial to shorten the course of the condition?

-   A Place the child in a steam-filled bathroom
-   B Administer inhaled budesonide
-   C Prescribe amoxicillin 125 mg tds for five days
-   D Administer inhaled salbutamol
-   E Prescribe paediatric cough suppressant containing codeine
-   F Administer inhaled tribavirin

Answer: *B*

MULTIPLE BEST ANSWER (MBA) QUESTIONS
In this type of question, a statement is given and is followed by a variable number of items. A specified number of these items are correct.

Example of a MBA question

A 65-year-old male smoker presents with a gradual onset of breathlessness on moderate exertion, and a cough with clear sputum. Chest examination reveals general reduction in breath sounds and the presence of a few rhonchi bilaterally. Spirometry reveals an FEV_1 of 50% predicted. Identify the THREE most appropriate therapeutic interventions to be considered following the British Thoracic Society COPD guidelines.

-   A Salbutamol inhaler
-   B Beclomethasone inhaler
-   C Ipratropium inhaler
-   D Salmeterol inhaler
-   E Sodium cromoglycate inhaler
-   F Oral theophylline
-   G Nebulised ipratropium
-   H Referral for long term oxygen therapy

Answers: *A C D*

EXTENDED MATCHING QUESTIONS (EMQ)

These typically consist of a scenario which has to be matched to an answer from a list of options. For any one item the candidate must choose one, and only one, of the options.

Example of EMQ

THEME: Reduced Vision

A	Basilar migraine	F	Occlusion of the central retinal vein
B	Cerebral tumour	G	Optic neuritis
C	Cranial arteritis	H	Retinal detachment
D	Macular degeneration	I	Tobacco optic neuropathy
E	Occlusion of the central retinal artery		

For each patient with reduced vision, select the single most likely diagnosis. Each option can be used once, more than once, or not at all.

1. A 75-year-old man, who is a heavy smoker, with blood pressure of 170/105, complains of floaters in the right eye for many months and flashing lights in bright sunshine. He has now noticed a 'curtain' across the vision of the right eye.   *H*

2. A 70-year-old woman complains of shadows which sometimes obscure her vision for a few minutes. She had felt unwell recently with loss of weight and face pain when chewing food.   *C*

3. A 45-year-old woman, who is a heavy smoker, with blood pressure of 170/110, complains of impaired vision in the left eye. She has difficulty discriminating colours and has noticed that her eye aches when looking to the side.   *G*

SUMMARY COMPLETION QUESTIONS
These are a fairly new type of question, which test candidates' critical reading ability from a summary of a paper presented in the question paper.

Example of a Summary Completion Question
The effects of obesity and weight loss on left ventricular mass and relative wall thickness: survey and intervention study

First read the extract from the Subjects and Methods section of the paper:

In total, 119 subjects from the city of Gothenburg and the surrounding areas were enrolled, comprising 61 men and 58 women with ages ranging from 37 to 61 years. The study population consisted of two groups of obese patients (body mass index 30–47 kg/m^2) and one group of non-obese subjects (body mass index 18–27 kg/m^2). The obese subjects were recruited from the ongoing Swedish obese subjects study, which is a nationwide trial designed to determine whether the mortality and morbidity among obese people who lose weight by surgical means differs from that in an obese reference group. The non-obese subjects were recruited from a randomly selected sample of adults living in the municipality of Mö Indal.

The two groups of obese subjects comprised 41 consecutive patients referred for weight-reducing gastric surgery (the 'obese operation' group) and 35 matched control subjects who were treated with conventional dietary recommendations ('obese control' group). The non-obese group consisted of 43 subjects matched with the obese groups for sex, age and height. Subjects in all three groups were examined again after one year. Four of the obese control patients were excluded from the study as they did not participate in the follow-up, leaving 31 subjects in the obese control group.

Body weight was measured with the subjects wearing light clothing and no shoes and was rounded to the nearest 0.1 kg. Height measurements were rounded to the nearest 0.01 m, and body mass index was calculated as the weight in kilograms divided by height in metres squared.

Systolic and diastolic (phase V) blood pressure was measured in the right arm using a mercury sphygmomanometer with the subject in the supine position after 10 minutes of rest. An appropriate cuff was used with the width at least 40% of the circumference of the arm. Echocardiography was performed on each subject in the left lateral decubitus position, using a commercially available ultrasound system (Accuson 128XP:Mountain View, CA) with 2.0–2.5 MHz transducers. Two dimensional echocardiography registrations were obtained with short axis and four chamber views. From the left ventricular short axis view, epicardial and endocardial perimeters were traced and mean wall thickness and cavity radius were calculated. Relative wall thickness was defined as the ratio of mean wall thickness to chamber thickness. Left ventricular mass was calculated according to the truncated ellipsoid algorithm from Byrd *et al.* Left ventricular diastolic volumes were estimated from the four chamber view, using the disc summation method (modified Simpson's rule).

All recordings were performed by doctors experienced in echocardiography, and 75% of the registrations were made by one investigator (IW). Each reading was assessed before statistical analyses took place, and only subjects with recordings of excellent or good quality were included in data analyses. As a result, 9 (13%) of the obese patients were excluded from the analysis of left ventricular wall thickness and mass and 20 (28%) from the estimations of left ventricular volumes. Only 1 (2%) of the lean subjects was excluded from data analyses because of deficient registrations. The standard error of a single determination of left ventricular mass among obese subjects was 17%, assessed by a double determination in nine patients.

Now look at this critique, which outlines the limitations of the design and method of the study.

Although the authors attempted to match the subjects carefully in each group for clinic (30)_____, this was neither a (31)_____, nor a (32)_____ study. Evaluation of obese subjects echocardiographically was (33)_____; this resulted in (34)_____ of patients and missing data which could have led to (35)_____ in the results. Only one blood pressure recording was taken; this may be (36)_____ of blood pressure over time and the lack of (37)_____ in measuring blood pressure in obese patients must cast doubt on the (38)_____ of the results. This could explain the relatively weak (39)_____ of changes in blood pressure and changes in left ventricular structure observed in the study. Other studies have (40)_____ the correlation between blood pressure monitoring and left ventricular mass.

For each of the numbered gaps in the critique choose one word from the following list which best completes the sense, marking the corresponding lozenge on your answer sheet.

A	association	**L**	reliability
B	bias	**M**	safety
C	blinded	**N**	selection
D	cohort	**O**	sensitivity
E	demonstrated	**P**	success
F	difficult	**Q**	typical
G	error	**R**	undertaken
H	exclusion	**S**	unrepresentative
I	precision	**T**	validity
J	questioned	**U**	variables
K	randomised		

Answers

30.	U	36.	Q
31.	C	37.	I
32.	K	38.	T
33.	S	39.	A
34.	H	40.	E
35.	B		

Areas to be Examined

a) Emerging knowledge

Keeping up to date is a very important aspect of personal and professional development. It is therefore essential that this is tested in the MRCGP examination. The questions will include articles which have been published in the preceding 18 months. Guidance to candidates is that current literature will be about articles that the 'average' General Practitioner would be expected to read. This means that questions will be drawn from the *British Medical Journal, British Journal of Medical Practice, Evidence Based Medicine* and *Drug and Therapeutics Bulletin.* Questions may also be asked about major trials that have had an impact on day-to-day patient management, for example 4S and UKPDS trials.

Candidates will not be expected to be able to remember details of the actual study design but the key messages from papers, and the evidence on which everyday clinical decisions are based will be tested. The questions should be answered in relation to the published evidence and not according to an individual's local arrangements.

The criteria for choosing the material are that it should:

- be relevant to current General Practice
- test the range of candidates' ability
- be a commons topic (recognised by the majority of General Practitioners)
- be an important topic (likely to change or impact on General Practice)
- require critical appraisal skills
- favour the well-read doctor

Example question

THEME: Hypercholesterolaemia

A   4S
B   CARE
C   LIPID
D   WOSCOPS

Match the most appropriate statement from these important papers on treatment of hypercholesterolaemia.

1.   Involved over 9000 patients and compared the effects of pravastatin with placebo in patients who had a MI in the past   *C*

2.   Pravastatin reduced the risk of stroke by 28% and the risk of fatal MI by 37%   *B*

3.   This trial involved 4444 patients   *A*

4.   This is a primary prevention trial studying the effects of treating hypercholesterolaemia   *D*

---

b)   Critical Appraisal

Critical Appraisal is an essential skill for all practising doctors and can probably be defined as the application of common sense, a questioning attitude and analytical thought in assessing the quality of information obtained from written material. Such material would include such things as research papers but also letters from hospital consultants or even something as straightforward as an audit or laboratory report. The formats of these questions will vary and there will be an increasing number of extended matching items or a short critique where the candidate has to 'fill in the blanks' by choosing from a menu of options.

c)   Statistics, Epidemiology and Research Design

Candidates are not expected to be expert statisticians as the examiners setting the papers certainly are not! A basic understanding of the commonly used statistical terms, including those used in evidence-based medicine is required. (Calculators are not necessary and are not actually allowed in the exam.)

EXAMPLE QUESTIONS

Results of Colorectal Cancer Screening Using Rectal Examination and Faecal Occult Bloods

Colorectal cancer

	Disease present	Disease absent
Screening +ve	120	60
Screening – ve	80	740

A	Has a sensitivity of 72%	F
B	Has a specificity of 92.5%	T
C	Has a positive predictive value of 60%	F
D	Has comparatively high sensitivity	F
E	The probability that a person with a negative test does not have the disease is approximately 10%	T

Electrocardiographic findings	Impaired left ventricular systolic function	Preserved left ventricular systolic function	Total
Abnormal	90	169	259
Normal	6	269	275
Total	96	438	534

Options:

A	$\frac{90}{438}$	E	$\frac{169}{259}$	I	$\frac{269}{275}$
B	$\frac{90}{275}$	F	$\frac{90}{259}$	J	$\frac{96}{438}$
C	$\frac{90}{96}$	G	$\frac{269}{534}$	K	$\frac{96}{534}$
D	$\frac{169}{438}$	H	$\frac{269}{438}$	L	$\frac{169}{534}$

Match item 1-4 below with the correct option A-L. Each option can only be used once.

1	Sensitivity	C
2	Specificity	H
3	Positive predictive value	F
4	Negative predictive value	I

THEME: Study design

A	Case-control study	D	Correlation study
B	Clinical trial	E	Descriptive study
C	Cohort study	F	Meta-analysis

For each study, select the most appropriate study design from the following letters options. Each option can be used once, more than once, or not all.

1. A survey is conducted to determine the prevalence of mitral valve prolapse and correlates of occurrence within the general population   *E*

2. The prior use of aspirin is compared among 500 patients with newly diagnosed colon cancer and 1000 healthy persons   *A*

3. Prevention of lung cancer in studies within a population of 12,000 smokers who are assigned randomly to receive either vitamin E and beta carotene or an inert substance   *B*

4. The reported national incidence rates of hepatitis B infection are associated with corresponding national mortality rates for liver cancer   *D*

5. The results of several investigations of exposure to environmental tobacco smoke and risk of lung cancer are combined to reach a summary conclusion   *F*

d) 'The Best Practice'

The main objective in this area is to identify if candidates are using current evidence on which to base their everyday clinical decisions. The format of these questions will usually be 'single best answers' using clinical vignettes. Although these are very time consuming to construct they are the most reliable way of testing candidates' knowledge. The examiners will develop these questions based on the best evidence which is currently available.

The single best answer questions usually consist of a description of a clinical scenario. The candidate will be required to select the best answer to the question. Other options may well be partially correct but there is only ONE BEST ANSWER. The best way to answer these questions is to read the patient description of each item carefully and be certain that you understand what is being asked. You should try to generate an answer and then look for that in the option list. It is important to read each option, carefully eliminating those that are clearly incorrect. Of the remaining options, you should select the one that you believe to be the most correct and mark it on the appropriate space on the answer sheet.

Example question

Stroke Prevention in Atrial Fibrillation
A 70-year-old man is found to have non-rheumatic atrial fibrillation, controlled on digoxin. He has had no significant previous medical problems. Choose from the list below the SINGLE best management on current evidence:

A   Aspirin 150 mg daily

B   Fixed dose combination of Warfarin and Aspirin

C   Dipyridamole 200 mg bd

D   Warfarin, with INR between 1.7 and 2.5

E   Warfarin with INR between 2.0 and 4.0

Answer: E

Reference: Stroke prevention in atrial fibrillation, Editorial BMJ 31 May 1997 and BMJ 24 May 1997.

HOW TO APPROACH THE MCQ-TYPE QUESTIONS

It is important to be aware from the outset that the scoring of all the stems is exactly the same irrespective of the format. Candidates are awarded one mark for each item answered correctly and marks are not deducted for incorrect answers or failure to answer. This encourages candidates to attempt all items.

It is important for candidates to read the stem carefully and each of its following questions individually in order to be clear about the question asked. Certain trigger words are used in MCQ-type questions and it is important to have a clear understanding of their meaning. These terms are reproduced in the introduction of the examination paper.

Trigger words used in MCQ-type questions:

- **Pathognomic, diagnostic, characteristic** and **in the vast majority** imply that a feature will occur in at least 90% of cases.
- **Typically, frequently, significantly, commonly** and **in a substantial majority** imply that a feature would occur in at least 60% of cases.
- **In the majority** implies that a feature occurs in greater than 50% of cases.
- **In the minority** implies that a feature occurs in less than 50% of cases.
- **Low chance** and **in a substantial minority** imply that a feature may occur in up to 30% of cases.
- **Has been shown, recognised** and **reported** all refer to evidence which can be found in an authoritative medical text. None of these terms makes any implication about the frequency with which the feature occurs.

Candidates are required to fill in an answer sheet by shading in a lozenge. A specimen of the marking sheet is shown on page 118. It may sound obvious but it is vital to ensure that the correct lozenges are filled in since the sheets are marked by computer and if you inadvertently fill in the wrong line of answers the score could be disastrous! If you wish to change an answer your mark should be erased as fully as possible and the new answer entered. Detailed instructions will be given at the time of sitting the examination.

Approach to Multiple Choice and Computer-Marked Questions

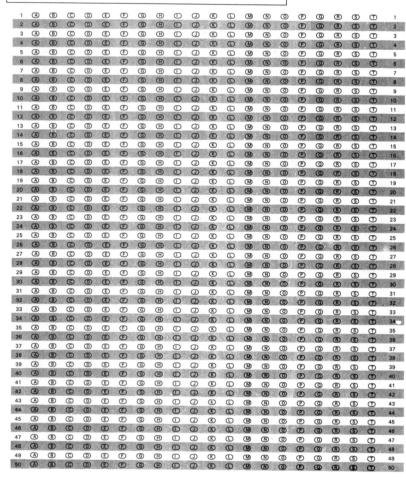

Design number 80301/A

Reproduced by kind permission of the Royal College of General Practitioners.

Having read the question you are faced with three possibilities:

1. You can answer the question. Good! Answer as you think best.
2. You are not sure of the answer but can use your knowledge and reasoning to work out an answer. Many of the questions will fall into this category and you may well be able to work out the correct answer.
3. You have no idea what the answer is. Because you do not lose a mark for a wrong answer – guess!

One technique is to work through the paper answering those questions that you are fairly certain about and then to go back to any questions you wish to think about again. Repeatedly going over questions you have answered can be counter productive, as answers which you were originally confident were correct may appear rather less convincing at a second, third or fourth perusal! In this situation first thoughts are usually best. Remember the examiners are not trying to trip you – they just need to find out how much you actually know! Don't try to look for hidden meanings, catches and ambiguities. Undoubtedly some people find MCQ-type questions easier than others. If you find this part of the examination difficult then practice more MCQs to improve your technique.

Revision for MCQ-type Questions

It would be comforting to read and learn a range of textbooks and articles and then feel confident in answering most of the questions. However, this is incredibly boring and time consuming! However, there are several methods to help you improve your scoring:

*   Practice as many MCQ-type questions as possible. There is a section of practice questions in this book. An excellent book, containing five mock examinations, is MRCGP: Practice Papers – 3rd edition by P. Ellis and R. Daniels (PasTest).
*   The RCGP have produced a set of interactive educational self-assessment programmes on two CD ROMs (PEP-2000), which have sample exam questions and are an excellent tool to identify strengths and weaknesses in your knowledge base. (Details available from RCGP website.)
*   Bear in mind the topic distribution and concentrate on these areas.

- After working through an MCQ paper it quickly becomes obvious which areas are your 'black holes' – concentrate on these areas. Many topics will not require extensive revision since you will already have developed the knowledge base required at medical school and through various other medical experiences.

Final hints

- The best way to obtain a good mark is to have as wide a knowledge as possible of the topics being tested in the exam.
- Read each question carefully and be sure that you understand it.
- Mark your responses clearly, correctly and accurately.
- Use reasoning to work out the answers and guess at those you do not know.
- Try to enjoy it and keep calm!

PRACTICE EXTENDED MATCHING QUESTIONS

Theme: Prescribing for patients in renal failure

A   Absolutely contraindicated
B   Higher doses may be needed
C   Monitor drug levels more often
D   No changes required
E   Reduce dose
F   Reduce dose frequency
G   Relatively contraindicated

For each drug below, choose the correct advice from the above list of options. Each option may be used once, more than once, or not at all.

1. Captopril in moderate renal impairment

2. Gentamicin in severe chronic renal impairment

3. Frusemide (furosemide) for pulmonary oedema in severe acute renal failure

4. Phenytoin in severe renal impairment

5. Cefalexin in severe chronic renal impairment

Theme: Over-the-counter medications

A   1% hydrocortisone ointment
B   Aluminium hydroxide/magnesium trisilicate
C   Aspirin
D   Chlorpheniramine
E   Loperamide
F   Loratadine
G   Malathion lotion
H   Paracetamol
I   Ranitidine
J   Should be investigated first
K   Sodium cromoglycate nasal spray
L   Topical clotrimazole
M   Xylometazoline nasal spray

For each patient below, choose the single most appropriate treatment from the above list of options. Each option may be used once, more than once, or not at all.

6.   A 24-year-old woman complains of vulval itching and a white vaginal discharge

7.   A 30-year-old man complains of heartburn, indigestion and reflux

8.   A 3-year-old girl is febrile and irritable with a generalised vesicular rash. She has a history of febrile convulsions in the past.

9.   A 21-year-old student suffers with hayfever. He is due to take his final exams.

10. A 54-year-old man has a two-month history of epigastric pain after meals

Theme: Prescribing for pain relief

A	Aspirin
B	Carbamazepine
C	Co-proxamol
D	Diclofenac
E	Ibuprofen
F	Morphine
G	Paracetamol
H	Topical ketoprofen
I	Tramadol

For each patient below, choose the most appropriate treatment from the above list of options. Each option may be used once, more than once, or not at all.

11. A 12-year-old boy has just had a dental extraction and is complaining of a painful jaw

12. A 70-year-old woman has bone pain from metastatic breast cancer. Simple analgesia has been ineffective.

13. A 65-year-old man has an acutely painful, red and swollen left knee. He has recently been started on bendrofluazide.

14. A 50-year-old woman has severe shooting pains in the left side of her face following an attack of shingles. She has tried a number of painkillers from the local pharmacist with no benefit.

Theme: Causes of vaginal bleeding

A	Atrophic vaginitis
B	Bleeding disorder
C	Cervical carcinoma
D	Cervical ectropion
E	Cervical polyps
F	Ectopic pregnancy
G	Endometrial carcinoma
H	Exogenous oestrogens
I	Foreign body
J	Normal menstruation
K	Spontaneous abortion

For each patient below, choose the single most likely diagnosis from the above list of options. Each option may be used once, more than once, or not at all.

15. A 20-year-old woman has a very heavy period and passes several clots. Her last period was 45 days ago. She is otherwise well.

16. A 22-year-old woman has been on the oral contraceptive for six months. She has developed intermenstrual and postcoital bleeding. Speculum examination shows the visible part of the cervix to be bright red.

17. A 78-year-old woman has had treatment for a uterine prolapse. She has recently developed vaginal bleeding which is increasing in severity. Uterine curettage reveals no histological abnormality.

18. A 34-year-old woman presents with dark vaginal bleeding. Prior to this she has had left iliac fossa pain for a few days. She has a history of pelvic inflammatory disease and irregular periods.

19. A 55-year-old post-menopausal woman has developed post-coital bleeding. She also describes dyspareunia and urinary stress incontinence.

Theme: Advice for travellers – vaccinations

A   All of G and yellow fever
B   All of H and meningitis
C   Hepatitis A and B, typhoid, polio, diptheria and rabies vaccines
D   Hepatitis A, typhoid and polio vaccines
E   Hepatitis A vaccine only
F   No precautions required
G   Rabies vaccine only
H   Typhoid and polio vaccines only
I   Typhoid vaccine only

For each traveller below, choose the correct advice from the above list of options. Each option may be used once, more than once, or not at all. Assume each patient is currently resident in the UK.

20. A doctor is travelling to Somalia to work for the International Red Cross

21. A businessman is going to a conference in Thailand

22. A 40-year-old man intends to travel to Barbados for a holiday. He had hepatitis A four years ago and received polio as a child.

23. A 12-year-old girl is travelling to rural France with her parents

Theme: Prescribing in pregnancy

A	Avoid in all trimesters
B	Avoid in first trimester
C	Avoid in second trimester
D	Avoid in third trimester
E	Avoid just before delivery
F	Avoid in more than one trimester
G	Continue treatment if already started
H	No restriction

For each drug below, choose the correct advice from the above list of options. Each option may be used once, more than once, or not at all.

24. Lisinopril

25. Warfarin

26. Phenytoin

27. Trimethoprim

28. Paroxetine

Theme: Causes of respiratory symptoms in children

A   Acute bronchiolitis
B   Asthma
C   Cardiac disease
D   Croup
E   Cystic fibrosis
F   Epiglottitis
G   Inhaled foreign body
H   Pneumonia
I   Respiratory distress syndrome
J   Tracheo-oesophageal fistula
K   Whooping cough

For each patient below, choose the single most likely diagnosis from the above list of options. Each option may be used once, more than once, or not at all.

29. A 2-year-old girl has been unwell for two months with difficulty breathing. She has a barking cough with no sputum. The cough is worse at night and after feeding. Sometimes the bouts of coughing end with vomiting. There is no wheeze.

30. A 3-year-old boy has a chronic cough for three months. He has had several chest infections and has required several courses of antibiotics. On examination he has a monophonic wheeze heard in the right lower lung field. He is systemically unwell.

31. A 5-year-old girl has been tired and irritable for a few days with a runny nose. She now has a cough and is wheezy. On examination her temperature is 37.8°C and she has nasal flaring, intercostals recession and cyanosis.

32. A 1-month-old baby has had a chronic cough since birth and has been treated for two episodes of pneumonia. He becomes cyanosed when feeding. He is on the 3rd centile for weight despite abdominal distension. When coughing, he produces copious amounts of secretions and appears to 'blow bubbles'.

Theme: Symptoms of cardiac disease

A	Angina
B	Aortic dissection
C	Aortic stenosis
D	Ischaemic cardiomyopathy
E	Non-sustained ventricular tachycardia
F	Paroxysmal supraventricular tachycardia
G	Sick sinus syndrome (trachy/brady)
H	Ventricular ectopy

For each of the patients below, select the most likely condition from the above list of options. Each option may be used once, more than once, or not at all.

33. A 19-year-old female describing rapid regular palpitations without loss of consciousness, primarily at weekends

34. An 82-year-old man with exertional chest pains and difficulty lying flat is admitted with an episode of syncope

35. A 55-year-old man, three months post anterior myocardial infarction with episodes of palpitations not associated with loss of consciousness

36. A 50-year-old woman with episodes of palpitations not associated with loss of consciousness and separate episodes of near syncope

Theme: Clinical trials

A	4S TRIAL
B	AIRE
C	HOPE
D	ISIS I
E	ISIS III
F	ISIS IV
G	LIMIT – I
H	RALES
I	SOLVD
J	WOSCOPS

For each statement, select the correct clinical trial. Each option may be used once, more than once, or not at all.

37. A primary prevention trial in hypercholesterolaemia

38. Has shown a mortality benefit in CCF patients taking spironolactone

39. Has shown the benefit of ACE I in patients with clinical signs of heart failure acutely post MI

Theme: Choice of contraception

A	Barrier methods
B	Combined oral contraceptive
C	Intra-uterine contraceptive device
D	Laparoscopic sterilisation
E	Levonelle 2
F	Progesterone depot injection
G	Progesterone-only pill
H	Rhythm methods
I	Vasectomy

For each patient below, choose the most appropriate management from the above list of options. Each option may be used once, more than once, or not at all.

40. A couple have had three children and are both sure that they have completed their family. The wife does not wish to take the oral contraceptive, as she is concerned about the possible risks, and they are not keen on using condoms. Both are aged 35.

41. A 25-year-old shift worker wishes to avoid pregnancy for at least the next six months. She suffers with regular classical migraines. Her partner has a latex allergy.

42. A 38-year-old married woman has had two children and would like to have reliable contraception. She is not absolutely sure that she and her husband would not want a third child at some stage.

43. A 21-year-old woman had unprotected intercourse at a party two days ago. She does not wish to become pregnant.

44. A 26-year-old Catholic couple attend their GP's surgery asking about contraception. The wife suffers from irregular periods that are painful and heavy.

45. A 28-year-old woman has discovered that her partner has been using intravenous heroin. She wishes to continue her sexual relationship with him.

Theme: Side-effects of medication

A	Amiodarone
B	Aspirin
C	Atenolol
D	Carbimazole
E	Chlorpromazine
F	Erythromycin
G	Co-beneldopa
H	Lisinopril
I	Lithium
J	Metformin
K	Sulphasalazine
L	Verapamil

For each list of side-effects below, choose the most likely causative agent from the above list of options. Each option may be used once, more than once, or not at all.

46. Cold hands and feet, fatigue, impotence

47. Peripheral neuropathy, pulmonary fibrosis, hyperthyroidism

48. Postural hypotension, involuntary movements, nausea

49. Thirst, polyuria, tremor, rashes

50. Sore throat, rash, pruritus, nausea

Theme: Anti-hypertensive medications

A   Amlodipine
B   Atenolol
C   Bendrofluazide
D   Bisoprolol
E   Doxazosin
F   Indapamide
G   Ramipril

For each patient below, choose the most appropriate medication from the above list of options. Each option may be used once, more than once, or not at all.

51. A 70-year-old lady with BP 190/80 and no significant past medical history

52. A 48-year-old businessman with type 2 diabetes mellitus and BP 160/95. Risk factors include ex-smoker, total cholesterol 6.4 and family history of IHD. Urine dipstix reveals proteinuria 1+.

53. A 50-year-old Afro-Caribbean man with long history of resistant hypertension currently receiving enalapril 20 mg bd, amlodipine 10 mg od and bendrofluazide 2.5 mg. What is the next agent of choice to replace one of the former?

54. A 40-year-old woman presents to casualty with a recent history of severe headache – she has a long-standing history of hypertension with poor drug compliance having stopped treatment for the past six months. Current BP 200/130. No focal neurological signs, grade 4 hypertensive retinopathy. Pregnancy test is negative.

Theme: The heart in systemic diseases

A	Acromegaly
B	AIDS
C	Ankylosing spondylitis
D	Endomyocardial fibrosis
E	Haemachromatosis
F	Sarcoidosis
G	Thyrotoxicosis

For each patient below, choose the single most likely diagnosis from the above list of options. Each option may be used once, more than once, or not at all.

55. An Afro-Caribbean woman with complete heart block and pulmonary hilar enlargement who returns to sinus rhythm after glucocorticoid treatment

56. A 30-year-old man with a dilated cardiomyopathy, diabetes and elevated liver enzymes

57. An African woman with a restrictive cardiomyopathy and elevation of a subset of her leukocytes

58. A 25-year-old man with a family history of Crohn's disease who has a second degree heart block

Theme: Hypopigmentation

A	Leprosy
B	Pityriasis alba
C	Pityriasis versicolor
D	Post-inflammatory
E	Vitiligo

For each patient described below, select the single most likely diagnosis from the list above. Each item may be used once, more than once or not at all.

59. A 5-year-old Asian girl presented with a few slightly scaly hypo-pigmented patches on her face for two months. She was born in the UK. There was a family history of thyroid disease but no history of similar skin problems. Fungal scrapings were negative. The lesions responded to 1% hydrocortisone cream.

60. A 23-year-old tourist from Brazil developed shooting pains in his right arm followed by clawing of his right hand. He had also noticed a reddish 5 cm patch on his right upper chest. On questioning it was revealed that the patch was initially whitish in colour. Histology showed granulomas in the dermis but stain for acid-fast bacilli was negative.

61. A 18-year-old Caucasian woman noted multiple hypo-pigmented patches on her upper arms and chest after a summer holiday in Lanzarote. Within a couple of months, she noted similar lesions on the backs of her hands. Although the lesions were asymptomatic she was quite concerned and asked her GP for a specialist opinion. The lesions were more prominent under Wood's lamp examination and scrapings for fungal examination were negative.

62. A 27-year-old Briton after a holiday in the Bahamas noted multiple hypo-pigmented patches on the arms and chest. Direct examination of the skin scrapings under microscope was described as spaghetti and meatball appearance.

Theme: Blistering in children

A   Bullous impetigo
B   Chickenpox
C   Chronic bullous disease of childhood
D   Epidermolysis bullosa
E   Staphylococcal scalded skin syndrome

For each patient described below, select the single most likely diagnosis from the list above. Each item may be used once, more than once or not at all. (

63. A 5-year-old boy had been unwell for three days with fever, coryza, runny nose and developed slightly itchy vesicles with clear fluid and surrounding erythema. His family members have been well and there was no history of foreign travel.

64. A child with atopic eczema developed multiple blisters with opaque fluid on his face and limbs. He was afebrile and otherwise well. His General Practitioner tried oral flucloxacillin and topical 2% mupirocin cream and the lesions subsided very quickly.

65. A 3-year-old girl presented with clusters of vesicles and bullae around her mouth and lower abdomen. She had been otherwise well and there was no prior history of herpes infection. Examination of oral mucous membranes was normal.

66. A 6-year-old girl presented with a history of blistering on her soles especially after walking. She also complained of sweaty hands and feet. Occasionally she had small blisters on her hands as well. There was no family history of note.

Theme: Leg ulceration

A	Arterial leg ulcer
B	Diabetic leg ulcer
C	Felty's syndrome
D	Squamous cell carcinoma
E	Venous leg ulcer

For each patient described below, select the single most likely diagnosis from the list above. Each item may be used once, more than once or not at all.

67. A 67-year-old diabetic man developed an ulcer on his right lower leg for three months and the size of the ulcer had increased since it was first noted. There was no history of trauma. The ulcer measured 2 cm in diameter, was crusted with an offensive smell and had a fungating appearance. A course of oral flucloxacillin made the ulcer slightly better.

68. A 76-year-old lady had a non-healing ulcer on her right medial malleolus for two years. She had a history of venous hypertension. She had had various creams, ointments and bandages without significant improvement. The ulcer became sore and weepy. She had been tested for diabetes and was negative.

69. A 52-year-old man with rheumatoid arthritis and an enlarged spleen developed painful ulcers on both medial malleoli for eight months. His rheumatoid arthritis had been under control with analgesics and sulphasalazine. On examination, the ulcer margins were well defined. The floor of the ulcer was clean and surrounding skin normal.

Theme: Dermatosis of palms and soles

A	Keratoderma
B	Palmoplantar pustulosis
C	Pompholyx
D	Reiter's syndrome
E	Syphilis

For each patient described below, select the single most likely diagnosis from the list above. Each item may be used once, more than once or not at all.

70. A 22-year-old man following an episode of urethral discharge developed joint pains, keratotic and pustular lesions on the palms and soles and inflammation of his glans penis.

71. A 24-year-old man originally from Zambia presented with hyperpigmented scaly lesions on the palms and soles. He was previously well and denied any recent medication. On examination he also had a few moist lesions over his perianal areas.

72. A middle-aged man had a long history of thickened palms and soles and recently developed dysphagia. Investigations showed that he had an oesophageal carcinoma.

Theme: Diabetic skin disease

A	Candidiasis
B	Diabetic dermopathy
C	Diabetic rubeosis
D	Granuloma annulare
E	Necrobiosis lipoidica

For each patient described below, select the single most likely diagnosis from the list above. Each item may be used once, more than once or not at all.

73. A 29-year-old woman with type 1 diabetes mellitus presented with multiple tiny asymptomatic dimples on both shins. The lesions had appeared over a couple of years. Her diabetic control was good.

74. A 16-year-old girl with type 1 diabetes mellitus had a slightly pruritic shiny yellowish red oval lesion on her right shin. She had tried topical steroids with no benefit.

75. A 14-year-old girl had a 3 cm diameter annular lesion with beaded margin on the dorsum of her right foot. Her General Practitioner had tried topical antifungals without any benefit.

Theme: Onycholysis

A   Dermatitis
B   Lichen planus
C   Psoriasis
D   Tinea infection
E   Trauma

For each patient described below, select the single most likely diagnosis from the list above. Each item may be used once, more than once or not at all.

76. A young woman was seen with thickened yellow-brown nails with distal onycholysis, affecting mainly her right hand. There were no nail pits and the patient did not have skin involvement. Mycology from an affected nail was negative.

77. A young woman was seen with onycholysis affecting her finger nails after she had started to work as a hairdresser. She had also developed an intermittent itchy rash affecting both palms.

78. A young man was referred with thickened nails and distal onycholysis. He had also noticed a patch of scarring alopecia.

Theme: Facial dermatoses

A	Acne vulgaris
B	Discoid lupus erythematosus
C	Kerion
D	Rosacea
E	Seborrhoeic dermatitis

For each patient described below, select the single most likely diagnosis from the list above. Each item may be used once, more than once or not at all.

79. A young man was referred with a pustular eruption on his cheeks. There was some background erythema. He also complained of gritty eyes.

80. A young man was seen with scaly erythema affecting his eyebrows with loss of some of the hairs.

81. A young man was referred with a pustular eruption on the right cheek over the beard area. The affected hairs were lost and the area appeared swollen.

Theme: Treatments for osteoporosis

A	Calcitonin
B	Calcium and vitamin D tablets
C	Cod liver oil
D	Oral bisphosphonate
E	Premarin
F	Prempak-C
G	Raloxifene

For each patient below, choose the single most appropriate medication from the above list of options. Each option may be used once, more than once, or not at all.

82. A 68-year-old lady who usually keeps very active was recently discharged from hospital following an admission for pain relief after a vertebral collapse. She underwent the menopause at 45 years. She is very keen to try and maintain her mobility and would like treatment.

83. A 48-year-old woman has been menopausal for the past three years. Her mother has recently been diagnosed with osteoporosis. She is concerned that she too will get osteoporosis and is keen for therapy.

84. A 40-year-old lady asks for advice regarding treatment and prevention of osteoporosis. She has quite severe asthma and over the years has required multiple short courses of oral steroids. A recent DEXA scan has been reported as within the normal range for her age. She is reassured by this but would like to try and prevent future problems if at all possible.

Theme: Infective diarrhoea

A   *Ascariasis lumbricoides*
B   *Clostridium difficile*
C   *Clostridium perfringens*
D   *Giardia lamblia*
E   Rotavirus
F   *Salmonella typhi*
G   *Schistosoma haematobium*
H   *Schistosoma mansoni*
I   *Staphylococcus aureus*

For each patient described below, select the single most likely infective agent from the list above. Each item may be used once, more than once or not at all.

85. A 19-year-old student returned from South America four months ago and complains of abdominal pain and bloody diarrhoea. On further questioning he remembers developing an itchy rash following which he developed a flu-like illness just before his return to the UK. On examination he has a 2 cm hepatomegaly and a colonoscopy shows several polyps in the descending colon, pus and blood.

86. A 50-year-old woman developed diarrhoea and vomiting several hours after dining out at a local restaurant. She attends her local casualty department. On examination she is not dehydrated but has mild abdominal tenderness but no local peritonism.

87. A 50-year-old man presents with a history of cough and diarrhoea to his GP's surgery. Before the results of any tests are available his GP is summoned to see him one week later and admits him urgently to the local hospital having made a diagnosis of acute small bowel obstruction.

Theme: Iron absorption

A	Chronic ITP
B	Chronic omeprazole (Losec) use
C	Coeliac disease
D	Excess dietary bran
E	GI bleeding
F	Type 1 von Willebrand's disease
G	Ulcerative colitis
H	Vegan diet

For each patient described below, select the single most likely cause for iron deficiency anaemia from the list above. Each item may be used once, more than once or not at all.

88. A 42-year-old Irish man with intermittent watery diarrhoea. He has a haemoglobin of 12.1 with a normal MCV and normal platelet count. In addition to a low ferritin confirming iron deficiency, the serum and red cell folate are also low.

89. A 72-year-old woman with early dementia and a prosthetic aortic valve. She lives alone but her diet is adequate due to meals on wheels. She is very tired but otherwise asymptomatic. Her full blood count shows a microcytic anaemia with a raised platelet count.

90. A 31-year-old woman who has suffered menorrhagia since her menarche. She has microcytic anaemia but a normal platelet count.

Theme: Vaccinations

A	BCG
B	Diphtheria vaccine
C	Heaf test
D	Hepatitis B hyperimmune globulin
E	Whooping cough vaccine
F	Yellow fever

For each type of vaccination below, select the single most likely vaccine from the list above. Each item may be used once, more than once or not at all.

91. Passive immunisation

92. Live-attenuated vaccine

93. Live bacterial vaccine

Theme: Causes of lymphocytosis

A   CMV infection
B   Erroneous laboratory result
C   Lymphoproliferative disorder
D   Non viral infection
E   Other reasons
F   Physiological

For each patient described below, select the single most likely cause of lymphocytosis from the list above. Each item may be used once, more than once or not at all.

94. A 20-year-old university student with cervical lymphadenopathy for two weeks and a negative Paul-Bunnell test.

95. A 45-year-old woman with night sweats and splenomegaly.

96. A 36-year-old man returning from Kenya with fever and splenomegaly.

97. A neonate with a haemoglobin at 11 g/dl and mild jaundice.

98. A 27-year-old woman with glucose-6-phosphatase deficiency treated with cotrimoxazole for a urinary tract infection.

Theme: Choice of inhaler devices for young children

A	Breath-actuated inhaler device
B	Dry powder inhalers
C	Metered dose inhaler
D	Metered dose inhaler + spacer
E	Metered dose inhaler + spacer and face mask
F	Nebuliser
G	Respirator

For each child below, select the most suitable device or combination from the above list of options. Each option may be used once, more than once or not at all.

99. Age 1–2 years

100. Age 3–5 years

101. With acute severe asthma

Theme: Aetiology of community-acquired pneumonia

A	*Chlamydia pneumoniae*
B	*Haemophilus influenzae*
C	Influenza virus
D	*Klebsiella pneumoniae*
E	*Legionella pneumophilia*
F	*Mycoplasma pneumoniae*
G	*Staphylococcus aureus*
H	*Streptococcus pneumoniae*

For each of the clinical scenarios given below, select the most likely organism from the list above. Each option may be used once, more than once or not at all.

102. A 35-year-old male presents two weeks after a flu-like illness with fever and productive cough. The chest X-ray shows evidence of cavitatory pneumonia.

103. A 70-year-old female presents with cough, rigors and confusion. On examination she has unilateral bronchial breathing and coarse crackles. Her chest X-ray shows unilateral lobar consolidation and air bronchograms.

104. A 29-year-old female presents with a three-week history of malaise, myalgia and cough productive of scanty, mucoid sputum. Chest X-ray shows multilobar consolidation.

Theme: The causes of wheezing

A   Asthma
B   COPD
C   Lymphangitis carcinomatosa
D   Pulmonary oedema
E   Sarcoidosis
F   Tumour
G   Vocal cord dysfunction

For each of the statements given below, select the single most likely diagnosis from the list above. Each option may be used once, more than once or not at all.

105. This diagnosis should be considered in patients with recurrent wheeze in whom pulmonary function tests are repeatedly normal and there is a history of multiple admissions and steroid prescriptions.

106. Unilateral wheeze in an elderly male who is a heavy smoker.

107. A 65-year-old female with bilateral expiratory wheeze, breathlessness and radiological evidence of pulmonary shadowing and mediastinal widening.

Theme: Causes of chronic cough

A	Asthma
B	Bronchiectasis
C	Bronchitis
D	Carcinoma
E	Fibrosing alveolitis
F	Foreign body
G	Habitual
H	Post-nasal drip
I	Reflux oesphagitis

For each patient described below, select the single most likely diagnosis from the list above. Each item may be used once, more than once or not at all.

108. An 18-year-old male with diarrhoea and an abnormal ECG.

109. A 40-year-old obese heavy drinker who is frequently woken with coughing bouts.

110. A 30-year-old with intermittent breathlessness and a nocturnal cough.

Theme: Models of the consultation

A	Balint
B	Byrne and Long
C	Helman
D	Pendleton et al
E	Stott and Davis

For each model of consultation, select the most suitable statement listed below. Each option may be used once, more than once or not at all.

111. Patients seek answers: to questions which include 'why me', 'why now'

112. Task orientated model broken into four key areas

113. Six phases to the consultation identified as a result of analysis of 2,000 tape recorded consultations

114. Described the pharmacology of the 'drug doctor'

115. Outlined seven tasks which taken together form aims for the consultation

Theme: Abnormal gait

A   Cerebellar disease
B   Lateral popliteal nerve palsy
C   Parkinson's disease
D   Sensory ataxia
E   Spastic paraplegia

For each patient, select the correct cause of abnormal gait. Each option may be used once, more than once or not at all.

116. A 65-year-old heavy smoker with nystagmus and a wide based unsteady gait

117. A 28-year-old patient with a steppage gait

118. A 76-year-old patient with a shuffling gait with non swinging arms

119. A 32-year-old with a stiff scissors gait

120. A 55-year-old who watches his feet and walks with a wide based stamping gait which worsens when asked to close his eyes

Theme: GMS payments

A   Deprivation payment
B   Designated area allowance
C   Inducement allowance
D   Initial practice allowance
E   Rural practice allowance

For each statement, select the correct option. Each option may be used once, more than once or not at all.

121. Paid to doctors setting up or joining a practice in a designated area for up to four years

122. Paid in three scales according to the Jarman index

123. Applies to doctors to setting up practice in an under-doctored area

124. Includes units for distance, difficult walking and blocked routes

125. Paid to GPs in sparsely populated areas with <1200 patients.

Theme: Autoantibody testing

A   Anti dsDNA
B   Cardiolipin
C   Gliadin
D   HLA b27
E   Intrinsic factor
F   Microsomal
G   Mitochondrial
H   Rheumatoid

For each of the conditions below, select the most appropriate autoantibody test. Each option may be used once, more than once or not at all.

126. Ankylosing spondylosis

127. Recurrent miscarriage and thromboses- antiphospholipid syndrome

128. Coeliac disease

129. Systemic lupus erythematosus

130. Primary biliary sclerosis

Theme: Welfare benefits

A	Attendance allowance
B	Disability living allowance
C	Disability Working allowance
D	Family Credit
E	Guardian's allowance
F	Incapacity benefit
G	Income Support
H	Unemployment benefit

For each statement, select the suitable welfare benefit. Each option may be used once, more than once or not at all.

131. For people working >16 hours per week bringing up children on low wages

132. A taxable benefit payable for up to one year if class 1 national insurance contributions have been paid.

133. Paid in the last six weeks of pregnancy and first two postpartum weeks to those unable to claim statutory maternity pay or maternity allowance

134. Has care and mobility components

135. Only applies to families taking on an orphaned child

136. Applicants must be working <16 hours per week and over 18 years of age

137. To qualify, the person must be over 65 years old

138. Conditions to be met include working at least 16 hours per week and the receipt of one other disability allowance to apply

Theme: Genetic conditions

A   Cystic fibrosis
B   Down's syndrome
C   Duchenne Muscular Dystrophy
D   Edward's syndrome
E   Klinefelter's syndrome
F   Neurofibromatosis
G   Pyloric stenosis
H   Spina bifida

For each of the statements below, select the correct genetic condition. Each option may be used once, more than once or not at all.

139. Inheritance is sex-linked recessive

140. Autosomal dominant inheritance

141. Often undetected occurs in 1/1000 live male births

142. The commonest trisomy

143. The commonest autosomal recessive condition

Theme: Skin disorders associated with Connective Tissue Disorders

A	Behçet's
B	Dermatomyositis
C	Discoid lupus
D	Rheumatoid arthritis
E	Systemic lupus erythematosus
F	Systemic sclerosis

For each of the scenarios below, select the most appropriate causative condition. Each option may be used once, more than once or not at all.

144. A 50-year-old female with multiple telangiectasia on her face

145. A 30-year-old female presenting with a butterfly rash

146. A 65-year-old with pyoderma gangrenosum

147. A 70-year-old male whose scaly plaques are not responding to treatment for psoriasis

148. A 40-year-old patient with genital ulceration.

149. A 75-year-old male who has a chronic cough and a rash on his fingers and around his eyes

Theme: Jaundice

A	Acute cholangitis
B	Acute gallstone obstruction
C	Alcoholic liver disease
D	Gilbert's syndrome
E	Hepatic metastases
F	Primary biliary cirrhosis
G	Viral hepatitis

For each of the following scenarios, select the correct cause. Each option may be used once, more than once or not at all.

150. 50-year-old female with gradual onset jaundice increasing pruritus who has a smoothly enlarged liver

151. 40-year-old female whose jaundice followed abrupt onset of right upper quadrant pain with a normal sized liver

152. A 60-year-old male who on examination is noted to have paucity of body hair and gynaecomastia.

153. 48-year-old male with right upper quadrant pain associated with rigors and dark urine

154. A 28-year-old male with an enlarged tender liver whose jaundice follows recent malaise and arthralgia

155. A 55-year-old male with a painless cholestatic jaundice and a palpably enlarged gallbladder.

156. A 30-year-old female with a normal liver, whose jaundice follows a recent upper respiratory tract infection

Theme: Mental Health Act (1983)

A	Section 2
B	Section 3
C	Section 4
D	Section 5
E	Section 37
F	Section 41
G	Section 136
H	None of the above

For each of the statements below, select the section of the Mental Health Act to which it belongs. Each option may be used once, more than once or not at all.

157. May be used to detain someone who is sexually deviant

158. May be used by a suitably qualified nurse

159. May be used by the police if the patient is in a public place

160. Allows for admission for assessment for up to 28 days

161. Covers the use of Community Treatment Orders

162. Covers periods of inpatient treatment up to six months

PRACTICE EMQ ANSWERS

Theme: Prescribing for patients in renal failure

1. **E**
    Captopril may become toxic if creatinine clearance is low. The risk of cardiovascular side-effects is greater. It is recommended that the starting dose is reduced and that the patient's renal function is monitored more regularly. ACE inhibitors are contraindicated in patients with bilateral renal artery stenosis or in unilateral renal artery stenosis supplying a single functioning kidney. Particular care should be taken in prescribing NSAIDs in combination with ACE inhibitors. Creatinine clearance in patients with renal artery stenosis may be well preserved and serum creatinine may be normal.

2. **C**
    Gentamicin excretion is very sensitive to reduction in renal function. It is also nephrotoxic, especially when given in combination with loop diuretics. Patients should have gentamicin levels monitored routinely. In renal impairment, monitoring should be more frequent and the dose will probably be lower.

3. **B**
    Frusemide acts on the loop of Henlé in the nephrons. Consequently, if the number of functioning nephrons are reduced, the dose of frusemide may need increasing accordingly to achieve the same diuretic effect. It is important to monitor renal function as it may deteriorate with the administration of any diuretic.

4. **D**
    Phenytoin is metabolised by the liver and is largely protein-bound in the blood. It is unaffected by renal function but may be affected by liver disease or co-administration of drugs that are also protein-bound.

5. **F**
    Most cephalosporins are excreted unchanged by the kidney and will accumulate in renal failure. Even in mild renal failure, some dose adjustment is required. In most cases, this means a reduction in dose frequency. It is often forgotten that renal function in older patients may be impaired even in the presence of a relatively normal creatinine.

Theme: Over-the-counter medications

6. L

Thrush may be treated with clotrimazole cream or pessary. Oral fluconazole is also available without a prescription (at a greater cost than the prescription charge).

7. B

Upper gastrointestinal symptoms in a young man are usually due to benign pathology. If the symptoms persist then a diagnostic endoscopy may be necessary.

8. H

The diagnosis is a viral illness, probably chickenpox. The most important treatment is to reduce her temperature to reduce the risk of a febrile convulsion. Paracetamol is useful as an anti-pyretic as well as an analgesic.

9. F

Several antihistamines are licensed for use in seasonal or perennial allergic rhinitis. Loratadine is a non-sedating antihistamine.

10. J

Epigastric pain of recent onset in a middle-aged (or older) patient requires medical assessment to identify those who are at risk of gastric carcinoma. There should be a lower threshold for diagnostic endoscopy.

Theme: Prescribing for pain relief

11. G

Simple analgesia, paracetamol and aspirin are appropriate for most mild pain. Due to its antiplatelet action, aspirin is probably not the best choice after dental extraction due to the increased risk of bleeding.

12. F

Simple analgesia is unlikely to be effective in malignant bone pain. Bone pain is likely to require strong analgesia and morphine, or similar, should be given. NSAIDs are also useful in managing bone pain and may be given in combination with opiates.

13. **D**

   Acute gout may be precipitated by diuretics. Pain is due to an intense localised inflammatory process and is best treated with potent anti-inflammatory drugs. If a patient is unable to take NSAIDs then colchicines or prednisolone are reasonable alternatives.

14. **B**

   Neuropathic pain following herpes zoster (or due to trigeminal neuralgia, amputation or peripheral neuropathy) is difficult to treat with conventional analgesics. Carbamazepine is of particular use in post-herpetic neuralgia. Other anticonvulsants such as gabapentin, sodium valproate and phenytoin may also be effective.

Theme: Causes of vaginal bleeding

15. **K**

   The most common cause of any period of amenorrhoea in a sexually active woman of childbearing age is pregnancy. If a patient was unwell or had ongoing bleeding, she should have an ultrasound and uterine curettage to exclude and treat retained products.

16. **D**

   The cervical canal is lined with columnar epithelium (which appears red) and the visible part of the cervix is lined with squamous epithelium (pink). The oral contraceptive increases the columnar zone so that it is visible around the cervical os, which is termed a cervical ectropion. Columnar epithelium is more friable, tends to bleed or produce mucus and is more prone to infection. If there is any doubt about the diagnosis then a smear and swabs should be taken.

17. **I**

   Post-menopausal bleeding should be assumed to be due to endometrial carcinoma until proven otherwise. Other causes include polyps, vaginitis and foreign bodies. Prolapse on its own rarely causes bleeding unless there is cervical erosion or infection. The most likely diagnosis is vaginal or cervical erosion due to a ring pessary that has not been changed.

18. **F**

   Pelvic inflammatory disease increases the risk of ectopic pregnancy due to blockage of one or both of the fallopian tubes. The history of irregular periods may have masked the amenorrhoea of pregnancy.

19. A

Atrophic vaginitis and vaginal dryness is common in post-menopausal women due to oestrogen deficiency. It may present with vaginal bleeding, dyspareunia, urinary infection, stress incontinence or prolapse.

Theme: Advice for travellers – vaccinations

Any traveller intending to visit a high-risk area should seek expert advice. Vaccination alone is not enough and travellers should also be advised to use insect nets and sprays and to avoid animal bites.

20. B

Sub-Saharan Africa has a high level of endemic infections and a broad vaccination programme is recommended. Many countries, but not Somalia, insist upon written proof of yellow fever vaccination.

21. C

South East Asia is another high-risk area. Sexually transmitted diseases are common and, apart from hepatitis B, there are no vaccines available as yet.

22. H

Travellers to the Caribbean are advised to have hepatitis A, typhoid and polio vaccinations. Childhood polio vaccination does not offer lifelong protection. Hepatitis A infection probably gives lifelong immunity and so this patient does not need vaccination against it, although it would do him no harm if there were any doubt.

23. F

Rabies has been eradicated from the United Kingdom but is still present in rural areas of other countries. The risk is small and rabies vaccine is not routinely given for travel to Western Europe.

Theme: Prescribing in pregnancy

24. A

ACE inhibitors are contraindicated in all trimesters of pregnancy. They cross the placenta and affect organogenesis and growth. They are associated with renal agenesis, renal impairment, oligo-hydramnios and skull defects.

25. F

Warfarin causes congenital malformations if given during the first trimester and fetal or neonatal haemorrhage if given prior to delivery. Warfarin is relatively safe in the second trimester, although some physicians favour the use of heparin throughout pregnancy.

26. G

Carbamazepine, phenytoin and sodium valproate are all associated with teratogenesis, particularly neural tube defects. These are more common with valproate. However, the risk to the mother and fetus due to uncontrolled epilepsy is greater than the risk due to the medication. Neural tube defects may be reduced by folate supplementation. Carbamazepine and phenytoin also increase the risk of haemorrhagic disease of the new-born, so both mother and child should receive vitamin K.

27. B

Trimethoprim is a folate antagonist and, therefore, has theoretical risks of neural tube defects if given in the first trimester. Penicillins and cephalosporins are not known to be harmful. Sulphonamides may cause haemolysis if given in the third trimester.

28. A

Manufacturers of SSRIs advise use only when the potential benefit outweighs the risk. There has been no evidence of teratogenicity with paroxetine although adverse effects with sertraline in animals have been reported.

Theme: Causes of respiratory symptoms in children

29. K

Whooping cough (pertussis) is rare in the UK. Pertussis vaccination is very rarely (<1/100 000) associated with severe brain injury and may cause epilepsy. The disease is often chronic and misdiagnosed as asthma or pneumonia. Absence of significant wheeze or fever and presence of lymphocytosis are suggestive. Complications include neurological damage, bronchiectasis and death.

30. G

Cough with wheeze is most often due to asthma. Localised, monophonic (single-pitched) wheeze suggests obstruction of a single airway. A common cause in young children is inhalation of a foreign body, often without any history to confirm this. Inhaled foreign objects are most likely to become trapped in the bronchus in the right lower lobe. A chest X-ray often makes the diagnosis.

31. A

Nasal flaring, grunting, intercostal recession, increased respiratory effort and cyanosis are all signs of respiratory disease in children and require urgent attention. In a child of this age, the most likely cause of respiratory distress is acute bronchiolitis. Diagnosis is largely clinical. The causative agent is nearly always respiratory syncytial virus.

32. J

Oesophageal atresia and tracheo-oesophageal fistulae may present immediately after birth with inability to feed. They may also present with failure to thrive, nasal regurgitation, recurrent aspiration pneumonia, cough or cyanosis. Passage of a naso-gastric tube is impossible.

Theme: Symptoms of cardiac disease

33. F

Some patients develop supraventricular arrhythmias at times of relative parasympathetic dominance (holidays, weekends) while others develop arrhythmias when the sympathetic system is activated (exertion).

34. C

The lack of symptoms such as syncope does not exclude the diagnosis of ventricular tachycardia and should be suspected in patients with ischaemic heart disease, particularly with a previous myocardial infarction.

35. E

Angina, dyspnoea and syncope are the classic symptoms of aortic stenosis. Syncope without palpitations can suggest a bradycardia as a cause , so suggesting the tachycardia/bradycardia syndrome if associated with separate palpitations.

36. G

Sick sinus syndrome is the most likely diagnosis in this patient. Although all the other conditions (excluding ventricular ectopics) can lead to loss of consciousness and syncope. Other clinical presentations are far more typical and common.

Theme: Clinical trials

37. J
38. H
39. B
WOSCOPS demonstrated 40 mg pravastatin od reduced the risk of non fatal MI by 31% and risk of death from all cardiovascular causes by 32% in hypercholesterolemia (LDL chol > 155 mg/dl). (NEJM 333:13cl–1307). RALES demonstrated a similar morbidity and mortality benefit (ie 30% reduction) using 50 mg spirono-lactone od, with ACE-I for heart failure ISIS 4 (Lancet 1995; 345;669–685) demonstrated 7% mortality reduction with captopril acutely (<24 h) post MI and failed to show any mortality benefit with magnesium or nitrate therapy in over 58,000 patients.

Theme: Choice of contraception

40. I
The most effective form of contraception is sterilisation of either the female or male partner. Vasectomy is preferable to female sterilisation as it does not require a general anaesthetic and the complication rate is lower. If there is any doubt, an IUCD provides good protection with minimal inconvenience.

41. F
Oestrogens are relatively contraindicated in women with migraine. IUCDs are not recommended in younger women because of their risk of infection and subsequent sub-fertility. Therefore her options are barrier methods, except her partner's latex allergy makes this difficult, or progesterone-only contraception. The progesterone-only pill requires good compliance and must be taken at the same time every day, which makes it less useful for shift workers. The progesterone depot injection is therefore most preferable for this patient.

42. C
The IUCD is probably the best form of contraception after sterilisation for an older woman in a stable relationship.

43. E

Post-coital contraception aims to prevent implantation in case of fertilisation. One option is Levonelle 2 within 72 hours of unprotected intercourse. The other option is insertion of an IUCD within five days.

44. B

The Catholic faith prohibits the use of contraception of any form. However, this does not mean that a Catholic cannot use contraception if they choose to do so. In this case, the combined pill will provide contraception and regular periods and may also reduce the amount of bleeding and pain.

45. A

Barrier methods will protect her against sexually transmitted viruses as well as pregnancy.

Theme: Side-effects of medications

46. C

The use of β-blockers is often limited by their side-effects. Fatigue and impotence, in particular, are commonly described.

47. A

Amiodarone is prone to cause many adverse effects, which limits the use of an otherwise versatile anti-arrhythmic.

48. G

L-Dopa-containing drugs often cause gastrointestinal disturbance, particularly nausea, which may be minimised by taking the tablets on a full stomach. Cardiovascular effects include postural hypotension, which may limit the dose that the patient will tolerate.

49. I

Thirst, polyuria, fine tremor and weight gain are common side-effects of lithium. Lithium may induce nephrogenic diabetes insipidus after prolonged usage.

50. D

Nausea and gastrointestinal upset are common, non-specific side-effects of carbimazole. Rashes and pruritus are also quite common and are allergic in origin. A patient who develops a rash on carbimazole should be changed to propylthiouracil. Agranulo-cytosis and neutropenia is a rare idiosyncratic reaction to carbimazole.

Theme: Anti-hypertensive medications

51. **C**
52. **G**
53. **E**
54. **B**
    Afro-Caribbean patients are often poorly responsive to β-Blockers and ACE-1 (low renin hypertension). Diuretics, calcium antag-onistics and doxazosin (αblockade) are often effective. Hyper-tensive emergencies, i.e. diastolic BP >120 mmHg, grade III/IV hypertensive retinopathy, renal impairment require admission.

Theme: The heart in systemic diseases

55. **F**
56. **E**
57. **D**
58. **C**
    Sarcoidosis is common in Black and Irish populations. Its commonest cardiac manifestation is through conduction abnor-malities, which may improve with steroid therapy. Permanent pacing is indicated. Hemochromatosis is a cause of dilated cardiomyopathy. It can also cause atrial fibrillation and ventricular arrhythmias. Endocardial fibrosis is a disease of equatorial Africa resulting in cardiac fibrosis and often-mild eosinophilia. Ankylosing spondylitis is strongly associated with HLA B27 (more so than Crohn's disease) and cardiac manifestations include conduction abnormalities and aortic regurgitation.

Theme: Hypopigmentation

59. **B**
    Slightly scaly hypo-pigmented patches on the face of children with atopy is a common disorder and more prominent in dark skin individuals. These are known as pityriasis alba which is a mildly eczematous (dermatitis) condition. The lesions usually respond to emollients and mild topical steroids can be added if required. Family history of thyroid disease is a red herring.

60. A

Hypo-pigmented and hypoaesthetic or anaesthetic patches are common findings in paucibacillary leprosy e.g. tuberculoid and borderline tuberculoid leprosy. However, in the type I leprosy reaction the typical lesions become inflamed and dysaesthetic. Along with skin, nerve trunks are well known to be involved in leprosy and could be the initial presentation of the disease. There should always be a high index of suspicion in patients from an endemic area for leprosy.

61. E

Vitiligo is a common disease affecting up to 2% of population worldwide. It is more common in younger people and a major problem in coloured skin population. In the white skin population explanation and cosmetic camouflage may be the answer but in the coloured skin population, potent topical steroids, phototherapy and surgical treatment in stable lesions may be contemplated.

62. C

Pityriasis versicolor clinically manifests as hypo-pigmented lesions and on microscopy typically shows a spaghetti and meatball appearance. Anti-yeast preparations like topical and systemic ketoconazole and oral itraconazole are useful. Although fungi are destroyed with treatment within a few weeks, the normal pigmentation may require a few months to recover.

Theme: Blistering in children

63. B

Chickenpox is common in children and is caused by varicella zoster virus. The virus stays in the dormant form in the dorsal nerve root ganglion and may cause herpes zoster in later life. The vesicles are centripetal in distribution. In adults, the infection can be severe causing symptomatic respiratory (viral pneumonitis) problems. Systemic anti herpes viral agents e.g. acyclovir are indicated.

64. A

Bullous impetigo is caused by *Staphylococcus aureus* and atopic individuals are prone to get secondary infections including bullous impetigo. Bullous impetigo responds well to oral antibiotics and general skin care is important to prevent recurrent infections.

65. C

Chronic bullous disease of childhood (CBDC) classically presents with clusters of vesicles and bullae around the face and lower abdomen. Skin biopsy reveals subepidermal blistering and IgA deposits. Sometimes the disease may continue into adulthood. Patients remain well systemically and respond to dapsone.

66. D

Epidermolysis bullosa (EB) mostly presents in childhood with increased skin fragility predominantly over trauma-prone sites.

Theme: Leg ulceration

67. D

Ulcers in diabetic patients result from venous and arterial causes and pyoderma gangrenosum, vasculitis and skin cancer need to be excluded. A short duration of the ulcer, increase in size and description of the ulcer would favour a diagnosis of squamous cell carcinoma, as in this case. Treatment requires complete excision.

68. E

History of venous hypertension and deep venous thrombosis, a long history and the typical site are important clues for varicose ulcers. Surrounding skin shows characteristic venous dermatitis. It is important to measure the ankle brachial pressure index (ABPI) and rule out any arterial component.

69. C

Presence of leg ulceration in Felty's syndrome is well recognised. Again it is important to rule out other common causes of leg ulceration. Treatment of leg ulcers due to Felty's syndrome may be difficult.

Theme: Dermatosis of palms and soles

70. D

This is a typical presentation of Reiter's syndrome. The heaped up keratotic pustular lesions on the palms and soles are known as keratoderma blennorrhagica and erosions on the glans penis are circinate balanitis. There no curative treatment for Reiter's syndrome.

71. E
History of genital ulcers in primary syphilis may not be spontaneous, as these are painless. Lesions of secondary syphilis are also asymptomatic. Primary and secondary syphilis is still seen in Asia, Africa and Latin America.

72. A
Patients with palmoplantar keratoderma (tylosis) may give a positive family history. A subgroup of them have an associated oesophageal carcinoma.

Theme: Diabetic skin disease

73. B
Diabetic dermopathy is a well-recognised condition and considered mainly a cosmetic problem.

74. E
Necrobiosis lipoidica is commonly seen in diabetics but can occur in non-diabetics as well. The lesions are largely asymptomatic and can rapidly enlarge in size or may ulcerate, requiring super potent topical steroids or intralesional steroids. Occasionally phototherapy may be beneficial.

75. D
Localised granuloma annulare and diabetes are uncommonly associated. It is important to rule out a dermatophyte infection which may mimic annular granuloma annulare. Asymptomatic lesions do not require any treatment and may burn out with time.

Theme: Onycholysis

76. D
The features could fit with psoriasis, lichen planus, dermatitis or tinea. The predominance of one hand and the absence of nail pitting and skin involvement makes a diagnosis of tinea infection more likely. Mycology is only positive in about 40% of samples.

77. A
The fact that her problem started after she gained employment as a hairdresser makes one think of an occupational dermatosis. With

the itchy palms, the most likely diagnosis is a dermatitic eruption, probably an allergic contact dermatitis.

78. B

The nail changes could be due to psoriasis, lichen planus or tinea. Lichen planus is more likely to present with nail and scalp signs, particularly scarring alopecia.

Theme: Facial dermatoses

79. D

The features could also fit with acne vulgaris but rosacea is more likely due to the eye involvement.

80. B

Seborrhoeic dermatitis and discoid lupus erythematosus can present with scaly areas within the eyebrows but in seborrhoeic dermatitis hairs are generally not lost.

81. C

Kerions tend to occur on the scalp but can infrequently occur in other hair-bearing areas. They tend to be unilateral. Rosacea can rarely affect one side of the face but the hairs are generally not lost and the affected site not swollen.

Theme: Treatments for osteoporosis

82. D

Oral bisphosphonates can improve bone mineral density. There are some people who are unable to tolerate them due to gastrointestinal side-effects. At the age of 68 the opportunity of hormone replacement therapy has really been missed. This prevents the dramatic decrease in bone mineral density that occurs at the time of the menopause. By delaying this fall to an older age the reduction in bone strength that leads to fracturing is also delayed.

83. F

This patient would be most suitable to start hormone replacement therapy. As she has an intact uterus it is essential to have both progesterone as well as oestrogen, this is the combination in Prempak-C. Premarin provides unopposed oestrogens which can lead to uterine carcinoma.

84. B

In the light of normal bone mineral density in a pre-menopausal woman there is no need for therapy, however adequate calcium in the diet is important and supplementation will have no deleterious effects (unless excessive quantities are taken).

Theme: Infective diarrhoea

85. H

S. mansoni is a trematode, which is found predominantly in South America, Africa and the West Indies. The intermediate host is the aquatic snail, which excretes cercariae (the infective form of the parasite) into fresh water. The cercariae penetrate the human bather's skin and cause a local inflammatory response (swimmer's itch). A flu like illness occurs acutely, which is characterised by fever, urticaria, eosinophilia, malaise, myalgia and diarrhoea. Clinical features apart from hepatosplenomegaly are lymphadenopathy and patchy pneumonia.

86. I

Staphylococcal food poisoning is characterised by an explosive onset of vomiting with a short incubation period of 6–12 hours in contrast to other bacterial causes of gastroenteritis.

87. A

Ascaris lumbricoides (roundworm) can grow up to 20 cm long and not uncommonly may cause small bowel obstruction at the ileocaecal valve. Other complications include acute appendicitis and obstructive jaundice from migration into the common bile duct. Pulmonary involvement occurs as a result of migration of larvae from the duodenum to the venous system. Expectorated larvae are swallowed and complete their maturation in the small intestine.

Theme: Iron absorption

88. C

Coeliac disease is not uncommon in patients of Irish ancestry and the combination of diarrhoea with iron and folate deficiency all point to malabsorption. Confirmation is by duodenal biopsy and by presence of anti-endomysial antibody.

89. E

A patient with a prosthetic aortic valve will be on lifelong warfarin therapy and warfarin control can be difficult in the elderly particularly if patients are intermittently confused about the doses of their drugs. Iron deficiency anaemia in elderly patients on warfarin is often related to gastrointestinal blood loss which is often occult. A modest rise in the platelet count may be seen in iron deficiency anaemia, particularly in a situation where the bone marrow is attempting to compensate for blood loss.

90. F

A history of menorrhagia since menarche is a strong clue to the possible diagnosis of von Willebrand's disease, an inherited condition, which produces bruising, epistaxis and menorrhagia. Type 1 is a mild form and is most common.

Theme: Vaccinations

91. D
92. F
93. A

Most bacterial vaccines including diptheria, cholera, typhoid and tetanus are killed vaccines, but BCG is an injection of live avirulent mycobacterium Bacille Calmette-Guérin. Viral vaccines including yellow fever, polio, measles, mumps and rubella are commonly live-attenuated vaccines. Passive immunisation is the transfer of antibodies and can provide protection against Hepatitis A, B, tetanus, rabies and chickenpox.

Theme: Causes of lymphocytosis

94. A
95. C
96. D
97. F
98. B

Even with a negative Paul-Bunnell test (used to confirm EBV infection), almost all transient lymphocytosis in young healthy adults is reactive to viral infections. Older patients with lympho-cytosis and other significant symptoms, such as night sweats and weight loss, must be investigated thoroughly for possible lympho-proliferative disorder or other underlying malignancies. Lymphocytosis can also be due to non-viral infective agents, such as malaria or tuberculosis. Lymphocytosis at birth is a normal finding. Rarely, nucleated RBC released during haemolytic episodes can be erroneously counted as lymphocytes by some cell counters.

Theme: Choice of inhaler devices for young children

99. E
100. D
101. F

The British Thoracic Society guidelines for the treatment of asthma reflect the trend for the use of a metered dose inhaler and spacer rather than a nebuliser for maintenance of children under 5. A facemask is added for very young children and for those who have poor co-ordination. Nebulisers continue to be used for acute attacks.

Theme: Aetiology of community-acquired pneumonia

102. G

When pneumonia develops after influenza infection the possibility of *Staphylococcus aureus* infection needs to be considered. The presence of cavitation although not specific to Staph infection would alert one to the diagnosis in the context of recent influenza infection.

103. H

There is good evidence to suggest the clinical presentation of pneumonia is a poor predictor of the likely aetiological organism, however *Streptococcus pneumoniae* is the commonest identified cause of community-acquired pneumonia and in an acute febrile illness with classic features of consolidation this would be the most likely aetiological organism.

104. F

The presence of community-acquired pneumonia in a young adult which has a gradual onset, constitutional symptoms and cough with scanty mucoid sputum would suggest the presence of infection by an atypical organism specifically *Mycoplasma pneumoniae*.

Theme: The causes of wheezing

'All that wheezes is not asthma'.

105. G

Vocal cord dysfunction is considered to be uncommon, however it is certainly underdiagnosed. This diagnosis should be considered when patients labelled as asthmatics, often with repeatedly normal pulmonary function tests, have a history of multiple admissions for severe exacerbations (but curiously good arterial blood gases) and a requirement for repeated steroid prescriptions. The aetiology is poorly understood and the confirmed diagnosis often difficult.

106. F

Unilateral wheeze should always alert to the possibility of a localised obstruction such as a tumour or less commonly a foreign body.

107. D

Lymphangitis carcinomatosa may produce wheeze and a chest X-ray resembling pulmonary oedema, however the additional presence of mediastinal widening due to lymphadenopathy or hilar lymphadenopathy should alert to the possibility of lymphangitis.

Theme: Causes of chronic cough

Chronic cough is a very common, disabling symptom in respiratory OP. The most common causes include previously undiagnosed asthma, post-nasal drip and reflux oesphagitis.

108. B

This is a young man with other symptoms and signs relate to bronchiectasis, the ECG abnormality relating to dextrocardia.

109. I

Obese men often have undiagnosed reflux oesphagitis.

110. A

This highlights the patient with episodic shortness of breath and nightly cough, classic of poorly controlled asthma.

All patients with continuing cough that is not settled with simple empirical treatments will need a bronchoscopy to exclude a foreign body or occult tumour.

Theme: Models of the consultation

111. C
112. E
113. B
114. A
115. D

Many analyses and descriptions have been carried out on the consultation. The four main categories describe whether the consultation is doctor or patient centred and whether the consultation is behaviour or task orientated. Task orientated, doctor centred models include those described by Stott and Davis and by Byrne and Long. The techniques described by Balint in *The Doctor, His Patient and the Illness* outline the use of transference and counter-transference in are an example of a patient centred, behaviour orientated model.

Theme: Abnormal gait

116. A
117. B
118. C
119. E
120. D

Cerebellar disease is most commonly a result of a tumour or demyelinating disease. Affected patients are unable to perform the heel–toe test. A high steppage gait suggests foot drop as a result of lateral nerve palsy, typically unilateral as a result of injury but may be bilateral in rarer disease e.g. Charcot-Marie-Tooth. Patients with sensory ataxia may be able to compensate to some extent for the lack of sensory input from the muscles in the lower leg by visual attention. Causes include subacute combined degeneration of the cord and cervical myelopathy.

Theme: GMS payments

121. D
122. A
123. B
124. E
125. C

The deprivation payment is classified as a capitation fee. The other payments are fees under Practice allowances. The Jarman index is used as a measure of deprivation.

Theme: Autoantibody testing

126.D
127.B
128.C
129.A
130.G

Ankylosing spondylosis may be diagnosed from a typical history examination and X-ray findings. HLA B 27 is positive in up to 98% affected patients. In coeliac disease 50% cases have a mild or moderate anaemia with a high MCV due to folate deficiency and testing for gliadin autoantibodies should be performed if the disease is suspected. 80% patients with SLE are positive for Antinuclear antibodies but the test may be positive in other rheumatological conditions. Double stranded DNA binding is more specific although present in only 50% cases. Mitochondrial antibodies are present in 90% cases with primary biliary sclerosis.

Theme: Welfare benefits

131.D
132.H
133.F
134.B
135.E
136.G
137.A
138.C

Income support, Family Credit and Disability Working Allowance are means tested. Attendance and Disability allowance normally only apply if the qualifying criteria are likely to be met for at least six months. Exemptions are made in the case of terminal illness. Attendance allowance is paid at day time and night time rates. In late pregnancy the maternity certificate is accepted as incapacity for work.

Theme: Genetic conditions

139.C
140.F
141.E
142.B
143.A

Duchenne muscular dystrophy affects males. Males with Klinefelter's are tall, thin, infertile and often intellectually impaired. Frequently the condition is unrecognised. Down's syndrome is by far the commonest trisomy. Cystic fibrosis has a frequency of 1:1600 live births.

Theme: Skin disorders associated with Connective Tissue Disorders

144.F
145.E
146.D
147.C
148.A
149.B

Systemic sclerosis results in tightening of the facial skin and multiple telangiectasia. The tips of the fingers lose their pulp and may develop infarcts. The gastrointestinal and pulmonary system is involved systemically. Pyoderma gangrenosum is associated with rheumatoid arthritis, Ulcerative colitis and Crohn's disease. The plaques of discoid lupus may be mistaken for psoriasis but do not respond to typical treatments for this. The classic triad of Behçet's disease is of oral and genital ulceration and uveitis.

Theme: Jaundice

150.F
151.B
152.C
153.A
154.G
155.E
156.D

Primary biliary cirrhosis typically affects females between 40–60 years and the onset of symptoms is gradual. Clinical examination of the patient with Alcoholic liver disease often reveals multiple dermatological signs which also include leuconychia, spider naevi and palmar erythema. Courvoisier's law states that in a jaundiced patient a palpably enlarged gallbladder is most likely due to malignant obstruction of the bile duct. In Gilbert's syndrome the jaundice is mild and often triggered by minor illness.

Theme: Mental Health Act (1983)

157.H
158.D
159.G
160.A
161.H
162.B

Sexual deviancy in itself is not covered by the Mental Health Act. The patient's mental disorder must be specified as either mental illness, severe mental impairment or psychopathy. Section 5 allows for the detention of a patient for up to six hours if the patient is already in hospital. Section 2 requires two medical recommendations and consent from an Approved Social Worker. Community treatment orders have been suggested as part of a new mental health act, and are not part of existing legislation.

PRACTICE SINGLE BEST ANSWER QUESTIONS

1. **A 24-year-old secretary has a four month history of palpitations when the 'heart misses a beat'. These episodes last a few seconds and are worse at night when she lays on the left-hand side. She is not obese and does not smoke cigarettes. From the list below select the single most likely diagnosis**

    ❏ A   Ischaemic heart disease
    ❏ B   Thyrotoxicosis
    ❏ C   Cardiomyopathy
    ❏ D   Anxiety
    ❏ E   Sick sinus syndrome
    ❏ F   Rheumatic heart disease

2. **Considering blisters in skin, indicate the ONE true answer from the list of statements below.**

    ❏ A   Bullous pemphigoid is a disease of middle age
    ❏ B   In pemphigus, the bullae are tense and haemorrhagic
    ❏ C   Dermatitis herpetiformis occurs in old age
    ❏ D   Both dermatitis herpetiformis and bullous pemphigoid have subepidermal bulla
    ❏ E   Treatment and follow-up can be stopped after a few months because pemphigus will 'burn' itself out

3. **A 58-year-old woman complains of generalised weakness. She was diagnosed as being hypertensive two months ago and has a blood pressure of 165/100 in spite of treatment with atenolol 50 mg daily. She is hirsute and obese with noticeable weight gain over the last 18 months associated with abdominal striae. Her fasting glucose is normal but she does have glycosuria++. From the list below select the SINGLE most relevant investigation**

    ❏ A   ESR
    ❏ B   Thyroid function tests
    ❏ C   24-hour urinary free cortisol level
    ❏ D   24-hour urine catecholamine
    ❏ E   Ultrasound scan of the kidneys
    ❏ F   Urea and electrolytes
    ❏ G   Random cortisol
    ❏ H   Fasting glucose

4. **When investigating malabsorption, which of the following is NOT a useful preliminary screening test?**

   - ❏ A   Microscopy and culture of stools
   - ❏ B   Faecal elastase concentration
   - ❏ C   Full blood count (FBC)
   - ❏ D   Mucosal biopsy
   - ❏ E   Erythrocyte sedimentation rate (ESR)
   - ❏ F   Immunoglobulins
   - ❏ G   Sweat test

5. **Which ONE of the following is an autosomal recessive disorder?**

   - ❏ A   Ichthyosis
   - ❏ B   Retinoblastoma
   - ❏ C   Myotonic dystrophy
   - ❏ D   Sickle cell anaemia
   - ❏ E.   Childhood blindness
   - ❏ F   Duchenne Muscular dystrophy

6. **A full-term infant develops jaundice on day three, which persists for the next two weeks. The liver function tests are normal except raised unconjugated bilirubin and the child remains clinically well. Select the SINGLE most likely cause from the following list.**

   - ❏ A   Galactosaemia
   - ❏ B   Breast milk jaundice
   - ❏ C   Sickle cell disease
   - ❏ D   Hereditary spherocytosis
   - ❏ E   Congenital CMV infection
   - ❏ F   ABO incompatibility
   - ❏ G   Biliary atresia

7. **Which ONE of the following drugs can be given to breast feeding mothers?**

   - ❏ A   Lisuride
   - ❏ B   Sumatriptan
   - ❏ C   Danazol
   - ❏ D   Digoxin
   - ❏ E   Tetracycline

8. **A 65-year-old man with atrial fibrillation present with right-sided tremor and giddiness. He has nystagmus on looking to the right and past pointing of the right hand. Which ONE of the following is the most likely diagnosis?**

☐ A   Wernicke's encephalopathy
☐ B   Parkinson's disease
☐ C   Right cerebellar infarction
☐ D   Multiple sclerosis
☐ E   Vertebro-basilar ischaemia

9. **Please indicate which of the following statements is NOT true. When considering recurrent miscarriage (loss of three or more pregnancies), it is recognised that**

☐ A   No cause is found in about 50% of cases
☐ B   Bacterial vaginosis has been shown to increase risk of miscarriage in the first trimester
☐ C   Parental chromosome abnormality is found in 15% of the couples
☐ D   Low dose aspirin has been shown to be beneficial in reducing miscarriage
☐ E   Polycystic ovary disease is associated with recurrent miscarriage

10. **A 58-year-old with rheumatoid arthritis and asthma complains of increasing breathlessness. Peak flows have steadily decreased over the last six months and are 70% of predicted. She takes salbutamol CFC inhaler PRN and beclomethasone 250 mcg bd. Choose the SINGLE most appropriate treatment from the following list:**

☐ A   Addition of long-acting β2-agonist
☐ B   Change inhaler device
☐ C   Increase dose of steroid
☐ D   Nebulised bronchodilator
☐ E   Intravenous steroid
☐ F   Leukotriene receptor antagonist

11. A 25-year-old secretary presents with a sudden onset of breathlessness and right pleuritic chest pain. Past medical history is unremarkable except for being diagnosed as Marfan's syndrome. Which ONE of the following is the most likely diagnosis?

- ❑ A Heart failure
- ❑ B Bronchiectasis
- ❑ C Pneumonia
- ❑ D Psychogenic
- ❑ E Pneumothorax
- ❑ F Pleural effusion
- ❑ G Anaemia

12. Select the SINGLE best answer from the following statements regarding tension headaches:

- ❑ A Are associated with aura in 10% cases
- ❑ B Is usually unilateral
- ❑ C Are more common in males than females
- ❑ D Is classified as chronic if occurring more than 15 times a month over six months
- ❑ E Codeine-based medication is most suitable for chronic headache

13. Which ONE of the following statements about genital chlamydia is not correct?

- ❑ A Is asymptomatic in up to 70% cases
- ❑ B Symptoms include intermenstrual and postcoital bleeding
- ❑ C The incidence of disease is stable
- ❑ D Patients can be screened by urinary PCR
- ❑ E Should be considered in females with right upper quadrant pain

14. Which single statement regarding smoking is NOT true?

❏ A   More than 10 million adults in the UK smoke
❏ B   10% 11–15-year-olds smoke at least 1 cigarette per week
❏ C   Approximately 70% smokers would like to stop
❏ D   20% smokers will be killed by their habit
❏ E   Nicotine replacement therapy doubles the rate of smoking cessation
❏ F   Bupropion increases the risk of seizure in at risk patients.

15. Regarding Attendance Allowance, which ONE of the following statements is true?

❏ A   Is unaffected by stays in hospital
❏ B   Is means tested
❏ C   Is paid at a flat rate
❏ D   A six month qualifying period applies unless the patient has a terminal illness
❏ E   There is no age limit

16. From the following statements regarding normal child development, pick the SINGLE correct answer:

❏ A   At 1 month, babies will vocalise and smile
❏ B   By 18 months, most children are able to get undressed
❏ C   At 6 months, most children can play pat a cake
❏ D   At 18 months most children are scribbling
❏ E   At 2 years the majority of children can stand on one foot

SINGLE BEST ANSWER QUESTIONS

1.   History of palpitations   Answer: D
The short duration of the 'attacks' are not suggestive of anything pathological. These are a normal occurrence and do not warrant investigations or treatment. Patients are usually more aware of these beats when they are stressed especially if they are thin. They occur more frequently if associated with alcohol and/or caffeine ingestion. Reassurance and lifestyle advice is all that should be 'prescribed'.

2.   Blisters in skin   Answer: D
In bullous pemphigoid, it is a disease of elderly, blisters are tense and haemorrhagic and histology shows subepidermal bulla. Dermatitis herpetiformis has subepidermal bulla but is a disease of young adult to middle age. Pemphigus occurs in middle age and has superficial flaccid blisters. However, it is a difficult disease to control and usually requires follow-up for many years while most cases of bullous pemphigoid will 'burn out' in one or two years

3.   Cushing's syndrome   Answer: C
This is a case of Cushing's syndrome. The fasting glucose is often normal but the glucose tolerance curve is usually diabetic and there is often glycosuria. It is a secondary cause of hypertension. A random cortisol is usually useless and the best screening test is the 24-hour urinary free cortisol

4.   Malabsorption   Answer: D
Fat globules in stools suggest malabsorption is likely; culture excludes infections. Low faecal elastase concentrations suggest pancreatic insufficiency. A FBC will alert to potential iron and folate deficiency; a differential may alert to specific diagnoses such as Wiskott-Aldrich syndrome (thrombocytopaenia), Pearson's syndrome (sideroblastic anaemia). ESR may suggest Crohn's disease while immunoglobulins screens for humoral deficiency and allows interpretation of coeliac serology. Sweat test screens for cystic fibrosis. Mucosal biopsy is not a preliminary screening investigation for malabsorption.

5. Autosomal recessive disorder   **Answer: D**
Sickle Cell anaemia (haemolytic anaemia) is an autosomal recessive condition. Ichthyosis (thick skin due to excessive keratin), Childhood blindness and Duchenne Muscular dystrophy (progressive muscular weakness) are X-linked. Myotonic dystrophy (myotonia with atrophy or degenerative changes in organs such as eyes, heart and gonads) and Retinoblastoma (malignant tumour of retina) are autosomal dominant conditions.

6. Jaundice   **Answer: B**
In breast milk jaundice, the child remains clinically well and the jaundice resolves with time.

7. Breast feeding mothers   **Answer: D**
Advisable only to give essential drugs to mothers. Lisuride may suppress lactation. Sumatriptan is present in milk – suggest withhold breast-feeding for 24 hrs. Danazol best to avoid due to possible androgenic effects in infant. Tetracycline is best avoided. Digoxin – amount is too small to be harmful.

8. Patient with atrial fibrillation   **Answer: C**
Nystagmus is more pronounced when the patient looks in the direction of the quick phase. All cerebellar signs are ipsilateral i.e. greater towards the side of the lesion. This is cerebellar nystagmus due to infarction because of atrial fibrillation – cerebellar lesion occur in multiple sclerosis but not in this case.

9. Recurrent miscarriage   **Answer: C**
Parental chromosome abnormalities have only been found in 3–5% of couples – the commonest being a Robertsonian translocation. Bacterial vaginosis has been reported to increase the risk of miscarriage two-fold.

10. Rheumatoid arthritis   **Answer: B**
Her arthritic hands may have some part in possible non-compliance and a breath actuated device may be more appropriate e.g. accuhalers, easibreathe

11. Breathlessness and chest pain   Answers: E

This is a case of primary spontaneous pneumothorax, which is common in Marfan's syndrome. It is caused by rupture of small bulla (caused possibly by congenital or inflammatory abnormalities) at apex of lung. This may because of the greater distance in these patients (who are usually tall) between the apex and base of lungs and hence slightly greater negative pressure at pleural space at apex.

12. Tension headaches   Answers: D

Aura only occurs in migraine headaches. Tension headache is more common in females and is usually bilateral, and the International Headache Criteria for chronic tension headache are given in answer D. Codeine should be used with caution due to the risk of rebound headache. NSAIDs, paracetamol and aspirin are effective treatments.

13. Genital chlamydia   Answer: C

Chlamydial infection accounts for up to 50% cases of PID and its incidence is rising. Chlamydial cervicitis causes unscheduled bleeding. Although relatively expensive urinary PCR is highly sensitive and specific and may useful in screening. At least 10 patients with PID develop a perihepatitis which may mimic cholecystitis.

14. Smoking   Answer: D

Approximately 50% of smokers will die as a result of their habit. Bupropion should be used with caution in anyone at risk of seizure.

15. Attendance Allowance   Answers: D

Attendance allowance is paid at a higher and lower rate depending on circumstances. It may be stopped while in hospital or residential homes. It is not means tested and is only paid to those over 65 years old.

16. Normal child development   Answer: D

Most babies do not smile or vocalise until 2 months. Getting undressed is usual by 2 years and standing on one leg by 3 years. Playing pat a cake is unusual before 1 year.

PRACTICE MULTIPLE BEST ANSWER QUESTIONS

1. **From the list, which THREE drugs have been shown to be of proven benefit for secondary prevention of acute myocardial infarction?**

    ❑ A   Atorvastatin
    ❑ B   Clopidogrel
    ❑ C   Dihydroperidines
    ❑ D   Amiloride
    ❑ E   Nitrates
    ❑ F   Beta-blockers
    ❑ G   Calcium channel blockers

2. **A 60-year-old smoker complains of a three-month history of retrosternal chest discomfort described as burning sensation, which radiates to the jaw. It is worse after food, and in cold weather. It is relieved with rest. There is no past history of asthma, diabetes, hypertension nor dyspepsia. Name the THREE most appropriate initial interventions.**

    ❑ A   Aspirin
    ❑ B   Antacids
    ❑ C   Ranitidine
    ❑ D   Clopidogrel
    ❑ E   Coronary angiogram
    ❑ F   Lifestyle advice
    ❑ G   Specialist referral

3. **Which THREE of the following statements about herpetic gingivostomatitis are true?**

    ❑ A   It caused by the type 2 herpes virus
    ❑ B   Is more commonly seen in adults than children
    ❑ C   May cause cervical lymphadenopathy
    ❑ D   Can be associated with fever and malaise
    ❑ E   Is usually associated with lesions on hands and feet
    ❑ F   Gradually resolves over a period of two weeks

4. **Which THREE investigations are most likely to aid diagnosis in a patient with a blood film showing macrocytosis?**

    ❑ A   Lead levels
    ❑ B   Folate
    ❑ C   Reticulocyte count
    ❑ D   Haemoglobin electrophoresis
    ❑ E   Thyroid function
    ❑ F   Magnesium levels
    ❑ G   Serum B12 levels
    ❑ H   G6PD activity

5. **Recognised features of tuberous sclerosis include which THREE of the following?**

    ❑ A   Petit-mal epilepsy
    ❑ B   Facial angiofibromatosis
    ❑ C   Periungual fibromata
    ❑ D   Retinal phakoma
    ❑ E   Skin depigmentation

6. **Which THREE of the following drugs should be avoided or used with caution in pregnancy?**

    ❑ A   Piperazine
    ❑ B   Simvastatin
    ❑ C   Frusemide
    ❑ D   Enalapril
    ❑ E   Chlorpheniramine
    ❑ F   Paracetamol
    ❑ G   Phenytoin

7. **A 25-year-old woman on the oral contraceptive pill has suddenly developed facial palsy associated with mild ataxia. Which THREE of the following are the most likely causes?**

    ❑ A   Stroke
    ❑ B   Ramsay-Hunt syndrome
    ❑ C   Multiple sclerosis
    ❑ D   Bell's palsy
    ❑ E   Otitis media
    ❑ F   Acoustic neuroma

8. A 45-year-old man with tremor of the outstretched upper limbs associated with sweating. Which THREE of the following are most likely?

❑   A   Cerebellar disease
❑   B   Anxiety
❑   C   Benign Familial tremor
❑   D   Alcoholism
❑   E   Hyperthyroidism
❑   F   Multiple sclerosis
❑   G   Wilson disease

9. Which THREE of the following are possible secondary causes of nephrotic syndrome?

❑   A   Non-insulin dependent diabetes
❑   B   Hypothyroidism
❑   C   Bronchiectasis
❑   D   Penicillin
❑   E   Diabetes insipidus
❑   F   Chronic infection

10. A 45-year-old asthmatic presents with night time wheezing and coughing, despite being on regular beclomethasone (dose of 400 mcg bd) and salbutamol PRN. He drinks 12 units per week and smokes 10 cigarettes per day. He is married with two children and a cat. Which THREE of the following options would be most appropriate?

❑   A   Leukotriene receptor antagonists
❑   B   Atrovent inhaler
❑   C   Avoid exposure to antigen
❑   D   Nebulised bronchodilators
❑   E   Advise to stop smoking
❑   F   Long acting b2 agonist
❑   G   Regular high dose inhaled steroids
❑   H   Intravenous steroids
❑   I   Inhaled sodium cromoglycate

11. **Free NHS prescriptions are available to patients with which THREE of the following conditions?**

☐ A   Thyrotoxicosis
☐ B   All patients with myasthenia gravis
☐ C   Hypo-parathyroidism
☐ D   All patients with diabetes
☐ E   Patients with colostomy
☐ F   Patients with hypertension
☐ G   Patients with asthma

12. **Which THREE of the following scenarios would suggest a ban of one month without driving (as set out by the DVLA)?**

☐ A   Following acute myocardial infarction
☐ B   After a stroke, which has completely resolved
☐ C   Severe asthma attack
☐ D   Syncope which has been identified and treated
☐ E   Epileptic seizure
☐ F   Following multiple TIAs
☐ G   Valvular heart disease
☐ H   Severe hypertension

13. **Which THREE of the following malignancies are associated with cigarette smoking?**

☐ A   Bronchus
☐ B   Bladder
☐ C   Breast
☐ D   Prostate
☐ E   Melanoma
☐ F   Cervix
☐ G   Colon

14. **Concerning alopecia identify the THREE statements below which are true**

☐ A   Tinea capitis is the commonest cause of temporary hair loss with scalp inflammation
☐ B   Post partum hair loss most commonly resolves spontaneously
☐ C   Alopecia areata only affects scalp hair
☐ D   Is a side-effect of thiouracil
☐ E   Hair loss associated with thyroid disease typically occurs in well circumscribed patches

15. **Tension headaches are a common cause of headache in general practice. Identify from the following the TWO statements which are correct.**

❑ A   May be triggered by viral meningitis
❑ B   Over 50% are unilateral
❑ C   Are equally common in males and females
❑ D   May be associated with aura
❑ E   Is described as chronic if occurring >15 times a month over a six month period

16. **Concerning DVLA regulations and group 1 entitlement identify the THREE correct statements.**

❑ A   The legal responsibility to inform the DVLA rests on the clinician who makes the diagnosis which affects a patient's ability to drive
❑ B   Following a myocardial infarction patients should not drive for a period of six months
❑ C   No driving restriction is required after a simple faint which has an obvious provoking cause
❑ D   A patient should not drive for one year following a first fit
❑ E   Insulin-dependent diabetic patients may be issued a driving licence if they retain recognition of hypoglycaemic symptoms

17. **Parvovirus B19 is a common cause of infection. According to Public Health Laboratory service information identify the THREE correct statements.**

❑ A   Causes a facial rash in children
❑ B   May cause hydrops foetalis
❑ C   Is a notifiable disease
❑ D   The peak incidence is in children aged 5–10 years
❑ E   In children is symptomatic in 80% cases

18. **Which TWO of the following statements concerning Bell's palsy are true?**

❑ A   Only affects the lower part of the face
❑ B   The 8th cranial nerve is involved in 20% cases
❑ C   May fail to resolve in 15% cases
❑ D   Treatment includes the use of high dose steroids unless contraindicated
❑ E   Once resolved the condition does not recur

19. Identify the THREE correct statements about Polymyalgia Rheumatica

- ❑ A   Causes limb girdle pain and morning stiffness
- ❑ B   Affects 15% patients over the age of 70 years
- ❑ C   Typically takes approximately four weeks to respond to steroids
- ❑ D   Is associated with temporal arteritis in over 5% cases
- ❑ E   In approximately 20% cases the esr is normal

20. Concerning PMS Practices which THREE of the following answers are true?

- ❑ A   Set-up costs are reimbursed
- ❑ B   Patients are to be able to access care from a GP within 24 hrs
- ❑ C   Practices are only required to make annual claims for payment of vaccination and immunisation services
- ❑ D   Are required to attain or make progress towards an 80% uptake of cervical smears in the screening age group
- ❑ E   Under PMS GPs are not exempted from CME and CPD

21. From the following statements on infantile colic select the TWO which are correct.

- ❑ A   Affects 80% infants
- ❑ B   Peaks in the 6–9 month age group
- ❑ C   Hypoallergenic formula milk has been shown to reduce crying
- ❑ D   Parents should be reassured the condition is harmless
- ❑ E   The drug of choice is dicyclomine which has a licence for children under 6 months

22. Which TWO of the following statements about Meniere's disease are true?

- ❑ A   Female patients are affected three times more often than males
- ❑ B   Typical symptoms are vomiting, otalgia and hearing loss
- ❑ C   Permanent sensorineural hearing loss occurs at an early stage of the disease
- ❑ D   Patients are required to inform the DVLA of their diagnosis
- ❑ E   Acute attacks should be treated with prochlorperazine or cinnarizine

23. **Concerning obesity identify the THREE correct statements from the following**

☐ A   Obesity is classified as a BMI greater than 40
☐ B   Is associated with an increased incidence of colonic cancer
☐ C   The Framington Heart Study showed an increase in mortality which directly correlated with weight gain
☐ D   The risk of developing type 2 diabetes is 40 times greater if the BMI is greater than 35
☐ E   Sibutramine reduces fat absorption by up to 30%

24. **Osteoporosis currently affects 1 in 3 postmenopausal women at an estimated cost to the NHS of £3/4 billion. Which TWO of the following are true?**

☐ A   A DEXA scan result showing a bone marrow density of 1 to 2.5 standard deviations below the mean is characteristic of osteoporosis
☐ B   The lifetime risk of a fracture after the age of 50 years in females is 50%
☐ C   A secondary cause for osteoporosis is identified in up to 15% affected females
☐ D   Bisphosphonates are the treatment of choice
☐ E   Menopausal smokers have a 50 % increased risk of fracture in old age.

25. **The Resuscitation Council of the UK issued new guidance for adult basic life support in 2000. Which TWO of the following statements are true?**

☐ A   The rate of chest compressions is 60 per minute
☐ B   If two or more persons are present the ratio of chest compressions to breaths should be 15:2
☐ C   Ventilation should be achieved by intubation
☐ D   If having checked for breathing there is no respiratory effort then chest compressions should be immediately commenced.
☐ E   For chest compression hands should be placed two finger breadths below the xiphisternum
☐ F   Chest compressions should depress the chest 4–5 centimetres

26. **Which TWO of the following statements about *Helicobacter pylori* are true?**

- ❑ A   Is associated with a 2–10 times increase risk of squamous cell carcinoma of the stomach
- ❑ B   25% of the population carry *Helicobacter pylori*
- ❑ C   Serological testing is limited by a sensitivity of approximately 60%
- ❑ D   *Helicobacter pylori* is a risk factor for short stature.
- ❑ E   The urea breath test has a specificity of approximately 95%

27. **A patient who is registered with the practice but has not been seen for three years presents on a Monday morning asking for a sick note. He tells you that he had the flu the previous week and was off work for four days. He has now recovered. Which THREE of the following statements regarding sick certification are correct?**

- ❑ A   A Med 3 may be issued in this instance as the patient was off sick less than 28 days
- ❑ B   When issuing a certificate for someone who is unemployed it should be completed based on their ability to do their last job
- ❑ C   A specific diagnosis must be given
- ❑ D   You cannot issue a Med 3 in this instance as the patient was not seen when ill
- ❑ E   No certification of any sort is needed for absences of less than 3 days
- ❑ F   A Med 5 form cannot be issued unless you have seen the patient personally
- ❑ G   It is against the terms of service for a GP to charge his patients for a private sick certificate

MULTIPLE BEST ANSWER QUESTIONS

1. Coronary Heart Disease prevention   Answers: A B F
Statins have been shown to be of benefit even when there is a normal cholesterol level and reduction of the baseline cholesterol of about 25% is recommended. Clopidogrel prevents activation of the platelet ADP receptor. The CAPRIE trial has shown that this drug is effective for secondary prevention of MI, stroke and peripheral vascular disease. However, aspirin remains the drug of choice for secondary prevention of MI. Trials are on going to assess if the combination of Clopidogrel and aspirin is better than aspirin alone. Beta-blockers are known to be of benefit in secondary prevention

2. Smoker with chest pain   Answers: A F G
This is suggestive of stable angina. Current guidelines suggest all newly diagnosed patients with stable angina should be referred when exercise stress testing will confirm the diagnosis and prognosis in angina. Coronary angiograms are not undertaken as initial investigations but reserved for when other investigations are inconclusive or where re-vascularisation is being contemplated. The NSF stipulates that such new patients are seen by a specialist within two weeks of referral. Lifestyle advice (e.g. stopping smoking, losing weight, exercise) is an important adjunct to therapeutic interventions, which include beta-blockers, sublingual nitrates for immediate symptom control and anti-anginal medication. Aspirin has been shown to be of benefit in stable angina and should be prescribed to all patients with Ischaemic Heart Disease.

3. Herpetic gingivostomatitis   Answers: C D F
It is caused by type 1; type 2 causes genital infections. Children are more commonly affected, often making them quite ill. They may cause drooling of saliva, pain, fever, malaise and cervical lymphadenopathy. Lesions on hands and feet would suggest hand, foot and mouth disease. It resolves over 10–14 days but some patients are so ill they require hospitalisation

4. Blood film showing macrocytosis   Answers: B E G
Common causes of macrocytosis include B12 and folate deficiency.

5. Tuberous sclerosis

Answers: B D E

There is no association with petit-mal epilepsy. Infantile spasms or myoclonic epilepsy presents in the neonatal period and may be difficult to treat. It is associated with learning disability. Facial angiofibromatosis develops in later childhood as a characteristic rash in butterfly distribution over the face, which can be treated by laser. Periungual fibromata are present in only about 5% of cases. Skin depigmentation most commonly present in the form of hypomelanotic macules.

6. Drugs in pregnancy

Answers: B D G

In the case of piperazine, there is no clinical evidence of harm but packs sold to the public carry warning to avoid in pregnancy except on medical advice. In the case of simvastatin, best to avoid since congenital anomalies have been reported, decreased synthesis of cholesterol possibly affects fetal development. With regard to enalapril, best to avoid since it may adversely affect fetal and neonatal blood pressure control and renal function. Also, possible skull defects and oligohydramnios. There is no evidence of teratogenicity with frusemide, chlorpheniramine and paracetamol. Phenytoin causes congenital malformations (screening advised); also caution in interpreting plasma concentrations – bound levels may be reduced but free levels are unchanged. It is wise to err on the side of caution and give only essential medication to pregnant women. See BNF for extensive list.

7. Facial palsy

Answers: A C F

Facial weakness can be seen as a rare complication of otitis media and in Ramsay Hunt syndrome. Bell's palsy is a common cause of acute lower motor neurone facial palsy. However, these syndromes would not be associated with ataxia. Multiple sclerosis is clinically defined as two or more episodes of neurological deficit occurring at different times and affecting different parts of the nervous system. The ataxia could be due to episodes of demyelination affecting the cerebellum and the brainstem. A haemorrhagic stroke is a possibility secondary to hypertension. Acoustic neuroma can affect the 5th, 6th, 7th and 8th nerves and the cerebellum. This may be hereditary as in Type 2 neurofibromatosis, which is autosomal dominant (chromosome 22).

8. Tremor of the outstretched upper limbs

Answers: B D E

Hyperthyroidism is associated with an exaggerated physiological tremor. Benign familial tremor is not associated with sweating.

9. Nephrotic syndrome   **Answers: A C F**

Patients can present as diabetic nephropathy with nephritic syndrome. There is no connection with hypothyroidism nor with diabetes insipidus. Bronchiectasis or other inflammatory diseases associated with amyloidosis can cause nephritic syndrome. Penicillin has no connection but rather penicillamine, gold or non-steroidal anti-inflammatories can be implicated in nephritic syndrome. Chronic infection or malignancy is another cause to consider.

10. Asthmatic with wheezing and coughing   **Answers: C E F**

Long acting β2 agonists e.g. salmeterol and eformoterol are useful in nocturnal asthma. It should be added to existing standard dose inhaled steroids, before increasing to high dose steroids. Leukotriene receptor antagonists (C4, D4, E4) e.g. montelukast and zafirlukast block effects of cysteinyl leukotrienes in the airways. They are sometimes used as adjunct to inhaled steroids in mild to moderate asthma. However would not rank in the top three interventions from the list. Avoidance of exacerbating factors is important to reduce severity of asthma. Smoking (passive or active) should be stopped. The common allergens are house dust mite, animal saliva (especially cat salivary antigen in fur) and pollens (especially grass). One could suggest a trial of pet removal or wash cat thoroughly every week to remove antigen from fur.

11. Free NHS prescriptions   **Answers: B C E**

Patients with thyrotoxicosis do not get free prescriptions but patients with myxoedema or conditions requiring supplemental thyroxine are exempt from the prescription charge. Patients with diabetes mellitus are also exempt from the prescription charge, except for those treated with diet alone. Patients with permanent fistula e.g caecostomy, laryngostomy or ileostomy needing continuous surgical dressing or appliance get free prescriptions. Similarly, patients with hypo-parathyroidism, hypopituitarism or continuing physical disability needing help of another person are exempt from the prescription charge. Finally, don't forget free prescriptions for pregnant women.

12. Driving ban   **Answers: A B D**
The DVLA (Driver and Vehicle Licensing Authority) sets out detailed rules regarding fitness to drive, which are updated almost annually. Following MI, unstable angina and bypass surgery it is recommended that patients do not drive for one month. The DVLA need not be notified. Following a stroke again one month is suggested. A fit after a CVA is considered to be provoked and does not extend the driving restriction. Following multiple TIAs three months is suggested. For a first true epileptic seizure one year and notification is required. Conditions such as asthma, diabetes, COAD do not require notification of the DVLA and no restriction exists unless they directly impair the ability to drive e.g. if associated with syncope or impaired vision etc. Congenital heart disease, valve disease, hypertension and conditions such as Marfan's carry no special driving restrictions. Complex rules exist for internal defibrillators and haemodynamically significant arrhythmias, which generally preclude driving.

13. Malignancies associated with cigarette smoking   **Answers: A B F**
Lung cancer is obviously very closely associated with smoking. Smoking also increases a person's risk of both bladder and cervical cancer. However, the risk of the other malignancies does not appear to increase with smoking.

14. Alopecia   **Answers: A B D**
Post partum hair loss (telogen effluvium) is common and caused by a temporary cessation of growth of hairs which enter the resting or telogen phase and most cases resolve after several weeks. Alopecia areata can affect any hairy skin including the eyebrows and beard. Alopecia due to thyroid disease is diffuse.

15. Tension headaches   **Answers: A E**
Tension headaches are commoner in females and are usually bilateral. Aura indicates migraine. The criteria for chronic tension headache have been defined by the International Headache study.

16. DVLA regulations   **Answers: C D E**
In accordance with GMC guidance the legal responsibility to inform the DVLA rests with the patient. Following a myocardial infarction driving must cease for four weeks. Simple faints do not require a period off driving but any unexplained collapse does require a period off driving for a minimum period of four weeks.

17. Parvovirus B19   Answers: A B E

Parvovirus B19 infection is also known as fifth disease or erythema infectiosum and typically causes a 'slapped cheek' rash on the face. In pregnancy parvovirus may cause hydrops and miscarriage.

18. Bell's palsy   Answers: C D

In Bell's palsy there is an idiopathic lower motor neurone palsy. This affects the upper and lower face distinguishing the condition from an upper motor neurone lesion which must be excluded. Other cranial nerves are not involved. Spontaneous resolution is unlikely to occur after 12 months.

19. Polymyalgia rheumatica   Answers: A D E

Polymyalgia rheumatica affects less than 5% adults over 70 yrs. A dramatic response to steroids is typical, usually in the first 2–4 days of treatment. There is association with temporal arteritis and these cases require high dose steroid treatment. The ESR is often normal and the CRP may be useful in these cases as it is usually raised.

20. PMS Practices   Answers: A D E

Set-up fees including accountants fees are funded by the scheme. Patients are to be able to access a primary care professional within 24 hrs and a GP within 48 hrs. PMS aims to reduce bureaucracy by minimising paperwork and claims. Services offered should enable the implementation of NSF, HImp and national cancer guidelines and practices are required to perform at least three audits per year to monitor achievement of key targets.

21. Infantile colic   Answers: C D

Colic affects between 10–40% infants and usually settles by 3–4 months. Dicyclomine is potentially dangerous and has no license for children under 6 months.

22. Meniere's disease   Answers: D E

There is no clear difference between the incidence in males/females. The classic triad is of vomiting, deafness and tinnitus. Some patients may complain of fullness in the ear. Hearing loss resolves between attacks early in the disease. On diagnosis patients should inform the DVLA. Once stable the DVLA may reissue their licence.

23. Obesity   Answers: B C D
A BMI greater than 30 is classified as obesity. Other cancers related to obesity include postmenopausal breast, endometrial and ovarian. In the Framington study the risk of death in 30–42 year olds was increased by 1% for every 0.45kg (1 pound) gained and by 2% in 50–62-year-olds. Orlistat reduces fat absorption. Sibutramine enhances satiety.

24. Osteoporosis   Answers: B E
A DEXA result between 1 and 2.5 SD below the mean is characteristic of osteopaenia. In up to 40% females and 60% males with osteoporosis a secondary cause (e.g. alcohol, steroids) may be found. HRT remains the treatment of choice even in established cases.

25. Resuscitation Council   Answers: B F
Chest compressions should be at a rate of 100 per minute. In basic life support mouth to mouth ventilation or bag and mask ventilation is used. If there is no respiratory effort two rescue breaths should be administered before proceeding to chest compression. Hands should be placed 2 centimetres above the xiphisternum.

26. *Helicobacter pylori*   Answers: B E
Helicobacter is associated with a 3–10 times increased risk of peptic ulcer disease and an increased risk of adenocarcinoma and the rarer MALToma. The various serological tests where compared in studies and all have a similar sensitivity of approximately 85%. The more expensive urea breath test has a sensitivity and specificity of at least 95%.

27. Sick certification   Answers: B D E
For absences greater than three days patients should self-certify. Absences over seven days require a Med 3 but this can only be issued if the patient has been seen, and can only be dated from that date. A Med 5 is issued when you have not seen the patient but another doctor e.g. in hospital has seen them. A Med 4 is used by the Benefits Agency for absences over 28 days. If you believe a patient is lying about illness an RM 7 may be sent to the DSS in confidence and they will arrange further review.

PRACTICE SUMMARY COMPLETION QUESTION

Reference

BMJ 1995; 311:1062. Dey, Collins, Woodman. 'Randomised controlled trial assessing effectiveness of health education leaflets in reducing incidence of sunburn'.

Reproduced by kind permission of the BMJ Publishing Group.

First read the extract from the Subjects and Methods section of the paper

The study population comprised holidaymakers travelling on Air UK Leisure flights from Manchester airport during August 1993. The unit of randomisation was the flight. Flights were stratified into long haul (North America and Jamaica) and short haul (Europe) and randomly allocated to the intervention or control arm. Before boarding, the health education authority leaflet *If You Worship The Sun, Don't Sacrifice Your Skin* was placed in seat pockets on flights in the intervention arm but not in the control arm. Cabin crew distributed questionnaires to passengers on Air UK Leisure return flights to Manchester. A history of sunburn was elicited by the question "Did you suffer from any sunburn during your recent holiday?" and, if so, whether this was associated with one or more of: redness of the skin, blistering of the skin, pain for less than a day, pain for more than a day. Adults completed the questionnaire for children. The study endpoint, severe sunburn, was defined as any episode of sunburn which was either painful for more than a day or resulted in blistering. Randomisation by group was undertaken to reduce contamination between the study arms. A clustering parameter was calculated for the study endpoint. Brier's adjusted was used for baseline comparisons, and 95% confidence intervals were constructed for the difference in proportions using methods appropriate to group randomised trials. Sixteen long haul and 62 short haul flights were randomised to the intervention arm and 15 long haul and 62 short haul flights to the control arm; 21,611 questionnaires were distributed and 14,956 (69%) returned. A total of 2,483 questionnaires completed by passengers who had not departed from Manchester airport during the study period and 88 inconsistent or illegible questionnaires were excluded from the analysis, leaving 12,385 evaluable questionnaires.

Now look at this critique, which outlines the limitations of the design and method of the study.

The authors used a   1   population flying from one UK airport but this population is likely to be widely   2   regarding possible   3   that may alter the response to the intervention. The use of a large   4   size and   5   tries to ensure that these   6   variables are evenly spread between the   7   and intervention groups. Stratification of the flights into long and short haul may lead to   8   since the geographical areas may be widely different regarding the potential for sunburn. The leaflet was placed in the seat pocket but it is uncertain whether this was read by the subjects or not. The   9   measure was   10   by questionnaire. No validated measures of outcome were obtained, leading to the possibility of   11   bias. Overall, the study adopts a   12   approach and this can lead to numerous potential causes of bias.

For each of the numbered gaps in the critique choose one word from the following list which best completes the sense.

❏	A	Confounding	❏	G	Study
❏	B	Sample	❏	H	Control
❏	C	Bias	❏	I	Outcome
❏	D	Self-reported	❏	J	Pragmatic
❏	E	Variables	❏	K	Heterogeneous
❏	F	Recall	❏	L	Randomisation

Answers

1.	G		7.	H
2.	K		8.	C
3.	E		9.	I
4.	B		10.	D
5.	L		11.	F
6.	A		12.	J

APPROACH TO THE ORAL EXAMINATION COMPONENT

A clear idea of the structure of the orals is essential for preparation for this part of the exam, as is an understanding of what is being tested and how. All assessment procedures flow better when the rules of the game are clear!

What is being tested in the orals?
The oral exists to assess areas of competence not tested in other parts of the examination. MCQ-type questions test factual knowledge reliably and extensively; hard facts and figures are not a part of the oral assessment. Similarly, appraisal and knowledge of the medical literature is tested in the written paper and detailed description of trials and papers should not be retested. Neither should the type of problem set in the problem solving-type component of the written papers be redebated. The oral has its own focus.

The aim is to assess the candidates' abilities to make decisions and justify the conclusions they reach, in the face of critical challenge from the examiners. Situations will be set or clinical problems raised which the candidate is asked to appraise.

It is important to understand this since demonstration of the decision-making process to the examiner is an essential part of the oral assessment.

An approach that analyses options and can look at the advantages and disadvantages of the possible solution before a final conclusion is reached, will inevitably gain more credit. A straightforward response such as: 'In this situation, I would without hesitation do this,' may seem decisive but may be viewed as rigid or dogmatic. The reasoning process is being examined far more than the ultimate decision is being judged.

For example, take the situation of an unreasonable out of hours call from a mother requesting a visit for her five-year-old son who has a sore throat. The examiner will not be awarding you marks for thinking 'This is the college examination and I must give the gold standard answer that I would visit without hesitation in case she was worried he had meningitis!' The ultimate decision 'to go or not to go' is not as highly weighted in the marking scheme as the candidate's ability to look at the options available and weigh up the pros and cons of each one before justifying a decision. Why is she asking for the visit? What are your on call arrangements? How well do you know her? How experienced are you as a GP? These are only some of the factors affecting the response. Decision-making is the process being tested with justification of any conclusions reached. There may be no black and white i.e. right or wrong answer: after all a lot of our working life operates in the grey area!

What is the structure of the orals?
There are two 20-minute oral examinations, each with two examiners. These occur consecutively with an approximate ten-minute break in between for changing tables.

In each oral, the candidate answers four or five questions. Both oral sessions are structured in the same way and both focus on testing decision-making skills in different situations. The topics to be covered are planned in advance by the four examiners. This ensures that the oral covers a fair range of General Practice subjects and that there is no overlap between the issues covered.

When meeting to plan the oral, examiners have no knowledge of the candidate's marks if other modules of the examination have already been taken. They cannot link their questions to the candidate's previous performance in any way. Thus the candidate will gain four individual and independent marks during the course of the orals. Marks can differ significantly between the two orals. Therefore during the break use the time to recover. Relax and put the previous experience behind you. Approach your second oral in a positive frame of mind.

After each pair of orals, the four examiners will meet to assess the candidate's marks and reach a final pass/fail decision.

What range of questions is asked?
The examiners plan the orals together to cover as wide a range of topics as possible. The aim is to create a fair examination by testing decision-making in as many different contexts as possible and avoiding repetition.

To do this a structure has been designed.

Three principal areas of assessment of the candidate's competence have been identified for testing in the orals:

- **Communication** This encompasses verbal and non-verbal communication techniques, skills for effective information transfer and principles of communication and consultation models
- **Professional values** This covers general moral and ethical issues, patient autonomy, medico-legal issues, flexibility and tolerance, implications of styles of practice, roles of health professionals and cultural and social factors
- **Personal and professional growth** This focuses on the candidate's personal approach to continuing professional development, self-appraisal and evaluation, stress awareness and management, burnout and change management

In order to focus and achieve a wide sample of questions these three competencies are tested in four areas or contexts relevant to General Practice:

1. The care of the patient specifically
2. Working with colleagues (Primary health care team and others beyond)
3. Society as a whole
4. Taking personal responsibility (for care, decisions, outcomes)

Questions testing each competency should focus on one of these four areas. Candidates should be aware of this structure as examiners may indicate, when phrasing a question, in which area they plan to mark.

Example:

Take the topic of diabetes, which can clearly be used to focus questions in many different ways:

The examiner may say:
'I would like to ask you a question looking at your communication skills.

How would you explain to an eighty-year-old patient that the nurse has found sugar in her urine and she probably has diabetes?'

In answering this candidates should focus on how they would use their **communication skills** with an individual **patient** in this age group.

Alternatively the examiner may say:

'I would like to ask you a question that focuses on your own personal development. You are concerned that you are becoming deskilled in managing diabetes since your partner took on responsibility for managing the practice diabetic clinic. What could you do about this?
This question is entirely focused on the candidate's **individual personal development** and the candidates should answer this at a personal level.

Alternatively the examiner may ask:

'I would like you to consider a situation which affects our professional values as a practice team. It is clear from your PACT figures that prescribing costs for blood glucose testing stix have significantly increased over the past six months. You have a new nurse running the diabetic clinic who is not following the practice protocol. What issues does this raise for you as a team?'
The approach to answering this question should be entirely different, concentrating on problems of differing attitudes and values which need addressing in managing a disease such as diabetes within a **multi-professional team**.

From the candidate's point of view it is clearly important to listen carefully to the question, to clarify it if you're uncertain what is being asked and to keep to the area in which the question has been focused. If it is an area in which you know very little and are performing poorly, you should say so and enable the examiners to move on to the next question where performance may be significantly better.

How is the oral marked?
Both examiners mark each question independently and at the end of the oral reach a final overall grade, exclusive of each other. Thus, over the two orals, four grades are obtained which are entirely independent of performance in any of the other modules.

The candidate's response is graded against a written scale. There are nine potential categories ranging from 'outstanding' through to 'dangerous.' The average passing grade is 'satisfactory.' To achieve this grade:

'A candidate characterised by a reassuring solidness rather than impressiveness. Able to justify only some approaches well, but most appear sensible. Adequate, not good decision-making skills.'

It follows that a spread of grading is achieved with the mean around the satisfactory level. 'Outstanding' and 'dangerous' grades are used only in extremely rare circumstances.

It is important for both examiners and candidates to recognise that each question must be structured in a way that will test a range of responses. They must enable the examiner to make a decision at the pass/fail level but at the same time have the capacity to test a candidate at merit level.

Recognition of this from the candidate's point of view is important for two reasons:

Firstly, as each question proceeds, it will get progressively more difficult and if the candidate is being examined well they will almost inevitably find there is a point beyond which they cannot deliver information. Thus they have reached their own personal level on the calibration scale and they will have no idea of this, beyond an uncomfortable feeling that they have not been able to stretch their answer to match the examiner's probing. This cannot be avoided. It is an examination. Thus even excellent candidates when stretched to the limit may feel they are performing poorly. It is crucial to come to terms with this feeling and not panic! It is intrinsic to the examination process.

Secondly, it may be equally difficult for a candidate at the pass/fail level to gauge their performance in the face of lack of any feedback from the examiners. The key is to take every question as it comes, approach each new one afresh and recognise that discomfort may be an inevitable part of the process.

Thus although the overall advice is to approach the oral as a professional interview and examiners are trained to make every effort to make the candidate feel welcomed and at ease, the discomfort and uncertainty of an examination process cannot be avoided.

When should I take the oral?
As the modular form of the examination has not run before, there is no data on which to base this answer at the time of writing. However, although the oral does not specifically test factual knowledge and

evidence-based practice, it can be seen that the process of decision making and justification cannot take place in a vacuum. A background of knowledge, awareness of the literature and experience of practice are required for you to justify your approach to decision making as a GP. Inevitably therefore the oral will be best approached towards the end of vocational training and with sufficient experience.

Helpful hints on approaching the orals
It is important to keep up to date. You do need to prepare for the oral. Working in pairs or as small groups can be stimulating. Questions can easily be devised and working out ways of increasing the difficulty of each question can be very educational.

The examiners are practising General Practitioners from all over the United Kingdom who have been selected and trained. Full understanding of all aspects of British General Practice is crucial. The oral will not focus on the candidate's area of practice but will expect a broad understanding of General Practice: for example an inner city GP could be asked about the problems of rural practice.

What happens on the day?
It is important to treat the event as one would any professional interview: dress smartly and allow plenty of time for travel. Candidates are briefed by the examiner marshal before the orals start. It is not a good idea to arrive at the very last minute.

All the examiners have been selected through an assessment procedure. The successful ones are then trained before they start examining. Candidates are not allocated to examiners from their own region of practice and should, for obvious reasons, not be examined by anyone they know personally. As the number of MRCGP courses throughout the UK expands, the situation occasionally arises where the candidate may have seen the examiner before. If the candidate recognises and would prefer not to be examined by them, a clear statement should be immediately made so that substitution can be arranged.

Observers may be present at the examination. Visitors from other medical faculties or professions attend to share and develop ideas for their own examination procedures. General practitioners interested in becoming examiners themselves observe for two days, before attending for the selection process, and experienced examiners may also observe for training purposes. The candidate should ignore any observer, as they are not contributing to the marking of the oral at all, only to the assessment of the examiners.

In addition a candidate may occasionally be made aware that a video camera is recording the oral, for examiner training purposes. Again, candidates are reassured that only the examiners appear on the screen and the tape is used entirely for feedback to the examiners concerned and for teaching purposes within the panel.

An example of a question sequence in an oral:

Question	Topic	Area of competence			Context			
		Communication	Professional Values	Personal & Professional Growth	Care of Patients	Working with Colleagues	Society	Personal Responsibility
1	Minor illness		√				√	
2	Asthma	√			√			
3	Re-accred-itation			√				√
4	Euthanasia		√		√			
5	Alcoholic partner	√				√		

Typical questions might be:

TOPIC 1 – MINOR ILLNESS

It could be said that in modern society, people are becoming de-skilled at handling minor illness. Why do you think that might be and what would you do about it?

As outlined on the above grid, this question is looking at our **professional values** as doctors in **society** and the candidate's decision-making process in designing strategies to tackle this problem.

The answer should focus on the reasons for the public's loss of confidence in handling minor illness, which of the factors are most relevant to the GP's professional practice and working values and how the problem could be tackled. The better candidate will also be able to reflect on the use of the term 'minor illness' and how decisions could be reached to redefine the term.

TOPIC 2 – ASTHMA

You decide a 3-year-old child, whom you have seen on several occasions with a dry cough, has asthma. How would you use your communication skills to explain the diagnosis to her mother?

This question is looking at the candidate's **consultation skills** and how decisions are reached in modifying them to explain the diagnosis in **the care of the patient**.

The answer should focus on eliciting the mother's understanding of the disease first before deciding what terms to use to explain the diagnosis at her level of understanding. The examiner might ask for the exact words the candidate would use and how he decided this. The question could extend for better candidates into the relevance of consultation models to this problem, which ones they might use and why.

TOPIC 3 – REVALIDATION

As you personally proceed with a career as a GP, how do you envisage future revalidation processes will develop and affect you as an individual?

This question is now in the area of ***personal*** responsibility for future professional growth through personal development plans and revalidation.

Candidates would be expected to explore how decisions might be reached on a revalidation programme and how this would fit with their own wants, needs and learning styles with reference to personal decisions to be made in pursuing their own education.

TOPIC 4 – EUTHANASIA

An 89-year-old patient of yours, bed-ridden with severe arthritis, asks you to honestly explain to her how many of the temazepam and phenobarbitone tablets stored in her cupboard she would need to take a fatal dose. What issues would this raise for you and how would you decide what to tell her?

This question is focused on ***professional values*** in ***the care of a patient***.

This question raises ethical issues relating to the legality of euthanasia balanced against truth telling and patient autonomy. Discussion of these would be relevant to the decision on how to respond professionally to this request. The examiner might expand the scenario by then suggesting that the patient was subsequently found dead in bed and the relatives are firmly against any thought of a post-mortem at her age. Further discussion of how to decide whether to inform the coroner or not and the ethical implications of the available options would be required.

TOPIC 5 – ALCOHOLIC PARTNER

Your health visitor asks to see you confidentially and reveals that several mothers have complained to her that your partner has alcohol on his breath even on morning visits. How would you respond to this?

This question deals with the competence area of ***professional values*** within the context of ***working with colleagues***.

Candidates should discuss the options open to them in dealing with this problem and the advantages and disadvantages of the various approaches with their inherent ethical issues. Awareness of the correct procedures for maintaining confidentiality while at the same time supporting the work interests of your colleague should form the focus of the discussion.

For further information on ethical problem solving please turn to Appendix 4, Ethical Problem Solving.

APPROACH TO THE ASSESSMENT OF CONSULTING SKILLS COMPONENT – VIDEO

In the past, the MRCGP examination has been criticised because there has been no assessment of clinical skills. The Royal College of General Practitioners has responded to this, and two approaches have now been developed – the video component and the simulated surgery.

The video recording is the normal method of assessing consulting skills for the MRCGP. Candidates have to submit a video recording of a sample of their recent consultations and this is accompanied by a completed workbook.

Preparing the video recording
Seven consultations need to be submitted, each lasting not longer than 15 minutes. Consultations lasting longer than 15 minutes can be submitted but the examiners will only assess the first 15 minutes of those consultations. All consultations must be conducted in English.

Candidates are required to include at least one consultation with a child under 10 years of age and at least one consultation with a significant social or psychological dimension.

Valid consent must be given by patients for their consultation to be video-recorded and the appropriate consent forms (provided in the college regulations booklet) must accompany the video and workbook. Detailed arrangement for consent and ethical guidelines are available in the publication 'Video Assessment of Consulting Skills Workbook and Instructions' which is available to all applicants and is obtained from the college. These ethical considerations also relate to the avoidance of physical examination of an intimate or sensitive nature and these must be conducted off camera. If these ethical guidelines and consent requirements are not adhered to, the video recording will be returned and deemed to be void.

The recordings have to be of sufficiently good sound and picture quality and if they do not achieve this standard they will be rejected. Again, detailed requirements for the choice of camera, sound recording equipment, camera positioning and lighting are given in the workbook and Instructions.

The Workbook
This contains the following sections:
*   The competencies to be demonstrated. This sets out the competencies that the candidate is asked to demonstrate in the recorded consultations.
*   Detailed instructions for recording consultations. This gives some practical advice about who should be recorded and how the recording should be made.
*   Video tape log. This acts as an index to the tape, to help the examiners locate particular points in the recording.
*   Consultation assessment forms. These are for the candidate's brief assessment of all recorded consultations.
*   Detailed evaluation forms. These are for the detailed evaluation of five consultations which the candidate selects for particular consideration by the examiners.
*   Ethical principles. These are the extracts from the RCGP's ethical guidelines on the recording of consultations.

How to approach the video component
After reading the ethical and practical considerations it is first of all important for the candidate to understand how the examiners approach assessment, so that the candidate has the best chance of succeeding. Consulting skills are a major element of professional competence for all General Practitioners. Competence has three attributes that determine the way it is assessed:
*   Competence is pre-defined. Candidates are given precise details about what the examiners are looking for. This is discussed later.
*   Competence is about outcomes not behaviours. There are many ways in which a doctor can arrive at the successful completion of a consultation. The examiners do not make the assumption that there is only one acceptable way of achieving this outcome, since this is highly dependent on the individual style of the doctor being assessed.
*   Competence is either present or absent. The examiners are judging whether or not the candidate has demonstrated competence in a particular situation. There is no measure of how well the candidate performs these specific competencies.

The Performance Criteria

Specific performance criteria have been developed, which candidates will either meet or fail to meet during the consultation. Assessment is achieved by collecting evidence and making judgements on whether or not these performance criteria have been met. It should be possible for the candidate, another doctor, or an examiner to watch a recorded consultation and decide upon whether or not the particular performance criteria were achieved.

Twelve of the performance criteria are preceded by (P) – these are the criteria which the examiners feel to be essential for a result of Pass in consulting skills. A further three performance criteria are proceeded by (M) – these are the criteria which the examiners feel must be demonstrated for a result of Pass with Merit in consulting skills. The examiners require at least three examples of each performance criteria out of the five consultations for a candidate to pass this module.

If satisfactory evidence of competence in all Pass level performance criteria has been found on at least three occasions in the first five consultations the tape will then pass. If sufficient evidence is not found then the next two consultations will also be assessed.

The performance criteria are as follows:

- **DISCOVER THE REASON FOR A PATIENT'S ATTENDANCE**

a) **Elicit the patient's account of the symptom(s) which made him/her turn to the doctor**

(P) PC: *the doctor encourages the patient's contribution at appropriate points in the consultation*
(P) PC: *the doctor responds to cues*

b) **Obtain relevant items of social and occupational circumstances**

(P) PC: *the doctor elicits appropriate details to place the complaint(s) in a social and psychological context*

c) **Explore the patient's health understanding**

(M) PC: *the doctor takes the patient's health understanding into account*

217

d)   Enquire about continuing problems

>   PC: *the doctor obtains enough information to assess whether a continuing complaint represents an issue which much be addressed in this consultation*

- **DEFINE THE CLINICAL PROBLEM(S)**

a)   Obtain additional information about symptoms and details of medical history

(P)   PC: *the doctor obtains sufficient information for no serious condition to be missed*

>   PC: *the doctor shows evidence of generating and testing hypotheses*

b)   Assess the condition of the patient by appropriate physical or mental examination

(P)   PC: *the doctor chooses an examination which is likely to confirm or disprove hypotheses which could reasonably have been formed OR to address a patient's concern*

c)   Make a working diagnosis

(P)   PC: *the doctor appears to make a clinically appropriate working diagnosis*

- **EXPLAIN THE PROBLEM(S) TO THE PATIENT**

a)   Share findings with the patient

(P)   PC: *the doctor explains the diagnosis, management and effects of treatment*

b)   Tailor the explanation to the patient

(P)   PC: *the doctor explains in language appropriate to the patient*

(M)   PC: *the doctor's explanation takes account of some or all of the patient's elicited beliefs*

c) **Ensure that the explanation is understood and accepted by the patient**

(M) PC: *the doctor seeks to confirm the patient's understanding*

• **ADDRESS THE PATIENT'S PROBLEM(S)**

a) **Assess the severity of the patient's problem(s)**

    PC: *the doctor differentiates between problems of different degrees of severity and manages each appropriately*

b) **Choose an appropriate form of management**

(P) PC: *the doctor's management plan is appropriate for the working diagnosis, reflecting a good understanding of modern accepted medical practice*

c) **Involve the patient in the management plan to the appropriate extent**

(P) PC: *the doctor shares management options with the patient*

• **MAKE EFFECTIVE USE OF THE CONSULTATION**

a) **Make effective use of resources**

    PC: *the doctor makes sensible use of available time and suggests further consultation as appropriate*

    PC: *the doctor makes appropriate use of other health professionals through investigations, referral, etc*

(P) PC: *the doctor's prescribing behaviour is appropriate*

b) **Establish a relationship with the patient**

(P) PC: *the patient and doctor appear to have established a rapport*

c) **Give opportunistic health promotion advice**

    PC: *the doctor deals appropriately with at-risk factors within the consultation*

Preparing the video recording and workbook for submission
Candidates are required to gather evidence of their competence, and the chosen method for this involves the making of video recordings of actual patients who consult the doctor in the course of the normal surgery, in the doctor's normal place of work. In addition a workbook is completed which involves reflecting on a selection of consultations, and committing these reflections to paper.

Candidates are allowed to choose which consultations they wish to present to the examiners so that they can show what they are capable of achieving if the consultation goes to plan. Allowing the candidate such a choice is to the candidate's advantage – a true impression of the candidate's consulting skills would require a large number of consultations to be viewed and this is obviously not feasible. The candidate is able to develop a 'mental picture' of what the performance criteria means, and is able to show a trainer (or other mentor) their work for confirmation that they have demonstrated competence. It is wholly unacceptable for the workbook to be completed by someone other than the candidate, but the candidate can be guided on how to produce the evidence of competence.

The video must include a range of challenging consultations that clearly demonstrate a candidate's consulting ability.

It is worthwhile initially to read a text which gives a good overall summary of the consultation process and which highlights the skills required for the doctor in the consultations. Two particularly useful books are *The Doctor's Communication Handbook* by Peter Tate, published by Radcliffe Medical Press and *The Inner Consultation* by Roger Neighbour, published by Petroc Press. After reading through these texts it should be clear what the various performance criteria mean and it should be possible to identify these performance criteria on a review of a particular consultation. The help of an experienced trainer, or mentor, is invaluable in helping the candidate to develop this self-assessment and reflection on their performance.

An example of a consultation and the highlighted performance criteria

Doctor   Hello Ian – what can I do for you today?

Patient   Well doctor – it's these pains in my stomach.

Doctor   Mmmm, please go on. (*Encourage patient's contribution.*)

Patient   Well – for the last three weeks I've had this pain in the centre of my stomach. It comes ands goes. It is worse first thing in the morning – that's also when I get some diarrhoea.

Doctor   Can I ask you a few more questions? [There is then a symptomatic enquiry, concentrating on the nature, frequency, relieving and exacerbating factors of the pain, also identical features about the diarrhoea. Enquiry is also made about having passed no blood or slime and whether the man feels well and his weight has been steady.] (*Encourage patient's contribution and obtain enough information for no serious cause to be missed.*)

I wonder if you have had any thoughts about these problems? (*Doctor takes the patient's health understanding into account.*)

Patient   I did read something about change in my bowels and indigestion in the newspaper and it said that I should see the doctor. I did wonder whether in fact it could be due to cancer or not.

Doctor   I see. Can I ask you a few more questions? I am not quite sure what job you do and whether there are any stresses or worries in your life at the moment. (*The doctor elicits appropriate details to place the complaint in a social and psychological context.*)

Patient   Well, I have had some worries at work with the recent merger. I am an accountant for the firm and the job is under threat of redundancy. My wife has just decided to give up work and she is now three months' pregnant.

Doctor   I see you look rather worried about that. (*The doctor responds to cues.*)

Patient   I am worried in case we can't manage financially. There is a mortgage to pay and the car loan – we both had such good jobs.

Doctor	May I examine your abdomen now please? [The doctor examines the patient's abdomen.] (*The doctor chooses an examination which is likely to confirm or disprove hypotheses which have reasonably been formed or to address the patient's concern.*)
	I have now examined you and I am pleased to say that I could find no abnormality. Your story sounds like a condition called Irritable Bowel Syndrome. When you are under stress the body produces extra adrenaline which stimulates the stomach and the bowels to cause the abdominal pain and the diarrhoea. (*The doctor appears to make a clinically appropriate working diagnosis. The doctor explains in language appropriate to the patient.*)
	I do not think it is cancer because there is no blood or slime in the motion, and your weight is steady and I could not find an abnormality. (*The doctor's explanation takes account of some or all of the patient's elicited beliefs.*) How do you feel about that? (*The doctor seeks to confirm the patient's understanding.*)
Patient	Yes, I agree, it does sound like Irritable Bowel Syndrome.
Doctor	There are several options. If you are not too troubled and worried we could just leave it to see if it settles. I could offer you some tablets to stop the spasm. If you do feel concerned still I could arrange for some further investigations. (*The doctor shares management options with the patient, the doctor's prescribing behaviour is appropriate, doctor's management plan is appropriate for the working diagnosis, reflecting a good understanding of modern accepted medical practice.*)
Patient	Well, I would rather have some tablets to relieve the pain.
Doctor	I will give you a prescription for some mebeverine. (*The doctor's prescribing behaviour is appropriate.*)
Patient	Thank you doctor, I will come back if there are any problems. (*The patient and doctor appear to have established a rapport.*)

Completing the video tape log

An example of the video tape log is shown on the following page. The function of the log is to allow the examiners to see at a glance the contents of the tape. For each consultation the start time, length of consultation and main reason for consultation must be documented. It is very important the log is completed legibly and correctly. Information about the outcomes of consultations and prescriptions used must be clear and exact to allow the examiners to make a fair assessment of these areas. Exact details on how the video tape log must be completed is found in the RCGP Workbook and Instructions to Candidates.

Consultation summary

For every consultation recorded, a consultation summary form must be completed. Each page is headed with a reference number, and this must correspond with the number used in the video tape log and on the patient's consent form.

This consultation assessment provides an opportunity to put each consultation into its proper context. As the recording is reviewed it is helpful to try to put yourself into the position of someone watching the consultation for the first time and who has no prior knowledge about the patient or the circumstances of the consultation. For example, the patient may be the local vicar and the various comments about religion may be quite normal, rather than religious paranoid ideas! An example of a completed consultation summary form is shown on the following page.

At the end of each consultation summary there is a rating for candidates to indicate the degree of perceived difficulty for the consultation.

CONSULTATION SUMMARY FORM

Reference number: 1

Consent for video-recording the above consultation
was obtained   Yes/No

Presenting complaint(s):   ***Abdominal pain and diarrhoea***

Relevant background information: ***Never seen before***
*(e.g. previous knowledge of or
consultation with this patient)*

Working diagnosis: ***Irritable bowel syndrome***

Outcomes of the consultation: ***Given prescription***
*(e.g. referral, no action,
certificate, review)*

Prescription: ***Given prescription for***
(provide full details of any   ***Mebeverine 135 mg tds***
*prescription given or test ordered,
with justification)*

In approximately 50 words outline the setting of the consultation, what
was achieved, and what issued may arise later.

***This patient had classical symptoms of irritable bowel syndrome which
were exacerbated by his recent stressful lifestyle. I managed to elicit
the patient's concerns about bowel cancer and could reassure him
appropriately. He has since returned to the surgery and his symptoms
have settled completely and his job is now secure.***

Summative assessment candidates
Please rate the degree of difficulty of this consultation by circling the
appropriate response:

straightforward/(moderate)/difficult

Helpful hints in approaching the recording and the completion of the workbook.

- Do not panic!
- Try to understand and be able to identify the key stages of the consultation process, linking this into the performance criteria that are required.
- Have a trial run first. Sit down with a trainer or mentor and work through a video-recording and begin to identify the performance criteria so as to be able to assess competence. Particularly, note any constructive comments made by the mentor or trainer.
- The commonest reason for failure of this section is the candidate not demonstrating shared management options with the patient.
- Finally, enjoy it!

APPROACH TO THE ASSESSMENT OF CONSULTING SKILLS COMPONENT – SIMULATED SURGERY

Simulated Surgery

The simulated surgery component of the MRCGP was developed as an alternative to the video component of the exam. It is designed to assess similar consultation skills to those that are assessed in the video. The simulated surgery is currently held twice a year but in the future it may become more frequent.

This module involves the candidate seeing a number of cases during a surgery (currently 12). Role players who are members of the public play the cases; they are not professional actors. Each candidate has a consulting station, which they stay in for the duration of the assessment. Each consultation lasts for 10 minutes and is separated by a 2-minute gap. After the first six consultations there is a 10-minute interval where simple refreshments are provided for the candidates. The exam is designed to be as similar to a normal surgery as possible.

Each candidate is given a running order for the surgery and a simple set of clinical records for each consultation. These records are necessarily brief and are normally no longer than one side of A4. There is nothing in these notes to mislead you. Each role player has an examiner who accompanies them and they assess you; your total marks are calculated by the independent judgements of 12 examiners.

Who is eligible to sit this module?
This module is currently available for candidates who have an insuperable difficulty in preparing videotaped records of their consultations. Common reasons that have been accepted so far have been:

- Moral or religious objections
- Not being in permanent practice
- Practising in an environment where a significant proportion of consultations are not conducted in English

Applicants from the Muslim community have most commonly requested the moral or religious exemption. Candidates from Saudi Arabia have so far provided the majority of applications in this group. Doctors working as locum practitioners make up the largest component of the second group. It is understandable that requesting to videotape consultations while working in this capacity may cause difficulties. The third group is available for practitioners who spend a significant amount of time not consulting in English. This includes doctors working in Welsh-speaking areas as well as those practising in communities with a high ethnic minority population.

If you feel that you may qualify to take the simulated surgery you will need to apply, in writing to the Convenor of the panel of examiners, stating your reasons. This letter should accompany your main application to sit the exam. It is a good idea to seek approval for this route of assessment at least four weeks before the closing date for the exam that you wish to sit.

What sort of case mix is there in a simulated surgery?

Each simulated surgery is made up of a variety of different cases. The aim is to assess areas of General Practice that are either common, or if less common, are important to manage well. A good example of this less common type is the breaking of bad news to patients. While we all hope that this will be an infrequent part of our professional lives, there is no doubt that such a situation needs handling with particular skill and sensitivity.

The age range is wide; so far there have been consultations with patients between the ages of 12 and 76. Children may be represented by consultation with their parents. There is an equal, or almost equal, balance between the sexes. Your skills in telephone consultation and in working with other members of the primary health care team may be assessed.

*Useful tip: so far there has **always** been a breaking bad news case. You would be well advised to plan for the exam with this in mind.*

The role players are not there to lead you astray or to trick you. If an answer is given there are no situations where they are instructed to change their history with further questioning. Where management is being discussed with a patient an initial reluctance to follow a suggested plan may be open for negotiation.

What are you allowed to examine?

There are no situations in this module which require any intimate examinations of a patient, such as gynaecological, rectal or breast examinations. If you do request to examine a patient because you feel it is appropriate, for example an abdominal examination, the role player is at liberty to decline. If a role player does decline any form of examination, including measurement of BP, you can assume that it is either not directly relevant, or if you had been able to carry it out, that the findings would have been entirely normal.

What sort of equipment do you need to take with you to the exam?

It is very important to remember that you should attend this exam well equipped. There will be no facility to supply you with items if you are not well organised. You will need to bring with you the following:

- A stethoscope
- A sphygmomanometer
- An auriscope and ophthalmoscope
- A patella hammer

Tongue depressors are provided.

The only form of written material that you are allowed to use in the exam is a copy of the British National Formulary (BNF). You are not required to bring one with you but you are strongly advised to do so.

What facilities can you assume that you have access to?

This is an exam set in British General Practice, in the context of the service provided by the NHS. You can assume that you have access to services normally available within this setting. For example you can assume that you can refer patients for radiological investigations, but that these facilities will be by appointment at a local hospital. You should not assume that there is an MRI scanner in your practice! You may assume that you have a normal, well equipped surgery and that you have easy access to other members of the Primary Health Care Team, along with facilities such as electrocardiography.

Standard members of the Primary Health Care Team that you may assume that you are able to involve include:

- Reception staff
- Practice managers
- Practice nurses
- District nurses
- Health visitors
- Attached social workers

You may also assume that you have a well-stocked library of patient information leaflets that are available at the reception desk following the end of the consultation.

You are also able to refer the patient to colleagues in secondary care where you feel this would be appropriate.

Blank prescription pads and medical certificates are provided. You may make notes while the consultation is underway. These notes do not currently form part of the assessment.

How are you assessed?
Unlike the video component there is a fixed marking schedule specific to each case. Each examiner compares your performance to this. The consulting skills that are assessed fall into one of five possible domains.

- Information gathering
- Doctor Patient interaction
- Communication
- Management
- Anticipatory care

Each case is marked using five individual constructs. Any individual case may be differently weighted for different domains. For example one case may contain two constructs representing Doctor Patient Interaction but have no marks awarded for pure information gathering.

In the first domain your skills at eliciting a history are examined. There is scope to do this by either taking a formal history or by giving the patient the space and consideration to tell their own narrative. This domain also includes gathering information from physical examination and from the records provided.

The second domain looks at skills related to putting a patient at their ease and developing a rapport. It is here that marks are also awarded for eliciting their ideas and concerns and for demonstrating empathy. This includes the use of both verbal and non-verbal skills. Showing respect for a patient's autonomy may also form part of the marking in this domain.

The third addresses communication skills. An example of this would be the appropriate explanation of an illness or a planned investigation in a way that the patient can understand. When producing an explanation for patients it is sometimes appropriate to write things down or to make very simple diagrams. Demonstrating an ability to share options with a patient is often assessed here, as are skills involving negotiation.

The fourth domain looks at skills needed to form a safe and effective management plan. These include using appropriate investigations, referral to specialists and prescribing. If you issue a prescription then the choice of drug and the dosage that you prescribe it in may form part of the assessment. Sensible use of time and resources may be examined in this domain.

The fifth, and final, domain is focused on anticipatory care. This often involves a process of 'safety netting'. In this process plans are made for follow-up where appropriate, involving input from the patient. Appropriate health promotion may form part of this component.

The consultation is a complex social interaction between a patient and a doctor. Any divisions or domains are by their nature artificial and act as a method for explaining the process of the consultation or as an aid to assessing it. There are some features that are common throughout though. A doctor who adopts a patient-centred approach to the consultation is more likely to arrive at an understanding of a patient's situation and their associated health beliefs. Being patient-centred means adopting an approach that puts the patient's thoughts and concerns at the top of your agenda. Once this is achieved it is easier to explain a problem to a patient in a way they are able to understand, taking into account their health beliefs. Once this understanding is achieved then sharing options and negotiating a plan becomes easier. This then naturally leads on to activity assessed in the fifth domain.

Anticipatory care involves two separate, but interwoven features. The first is the doctor's understanding of the natural history of a condition or situation, and in particular an appreciation of the risks, either physical or psychological that a patient may encounter following the end of the consultation. The second requires an understanding of a patient's ideas, concerns and expectations. Both of these elements need to be addressed to 'enable' the patient and to help them to face the future.

Useful tip: in addition to finding out why you think a patient has attended always try to find out what the patient's perceptions or fears may be about the situation.

Each construct is marked by the examiner based on a shortened version of the oral marking grades.

- G (good) 5 marks
- S (satisfactory) 4 marks
- B (borderline) 3 marks
- N (not very good) 2 marks
- P (poor) 1 mark
- U (unacceptable) 0 marks
- (omitted) 0 marks

How are the pass and merit marks calculated?

When the exam is over the examiners carry out an exercise to set the pass and merit marks. This takes into account the overall performance of candidates. There is not a requirement to pass a certain number of consultations but to perform overall to an acceptable standard. It is likely that in the future there will also be a requirement to perform to a certain overall standard in each domain.

The following is an example of a case that reflects a relatively low challenge situation in General Practice.

TOPIC OF CASE:	**ALLERGIC RHINITIS**
Suggested name for patient:	**Megan Hope**
Age:	**22**
Sex:	**Female**

ROLE PLAYER BRIEFING:

Opening statement: *'I seem to have a blocked and runny nose, doctor'*

Allow the doctor to ask questions about your blocked nose, and find out from your replies that:

- It has been getting increasingly worse
- It has been present for about two months and is not getting any better
- It started after you moved to a dusty old house
- You have not felt unwell
- You have no cough, hoarseness or headache. You have not taken your temperature.
- You have not stopped work/college or stayed in bed
- You have taken some decongestants but they haven't helped much
- You had a sore throat, which was treated with penicillin, six months ago

You should expect to have your nose and/or throat examined. If either of these actions is not performed gently, show some discomfort.

The doctor should know from your records that you had severe sinusitis two years ago and were ill for three weeks. You felt exceptionally unwell. One of your concerns, which you should reveal if the subject is raised, is that this nasal congestion might be sinusitis coming back again.

Another concern is that you are anxious to be well for a special social event in four days' time (e.g. bridesmaid at family wedding). You would not normally have come for a blocked nose, but hope that treating it would clear it up before the wedding. This concern should be voiced if the doctor prompts for it in any way (e.g. 'Why have you come now?' or 'Is there anything else that worries you about it?').

You are expecting to receive antibiotics, but will be content to receive an explanation as to why they are not necessary. If offered a prescription for antibiotics you will accept it. If asked, you are not allergic to any antibiotics. If the diagnosis of allergic rhinitis is made then you want to know: allergic to what?; what can be done to find out?; what can be done to treat it?. If you are offered a choice between taking an anti-histamine or using a nasal spray ask for an explanation of the pros and cons. Make your choice dependent on the explanation.

Simulated Surgery

RECORDS

Name:	Megan Hope
Age:	22
Sex:	Female
2 years ago:	Severe Sinusitis Rx Doxycycline
	Off work – 3 weeks
6 months ago:	Sore throat – Rx Penicillin V.

NAME :   **Megan Hope**   **EXAMINER :**

EXAM CASE: **STATION:**   **CANDIDATE NO:**

---

1. **Information gathering – Interview/history taking**

   Good
   i) Clarifies history of blocked nose, duration, etc.
   ii) Establishes patient's self-management up to now
   iii) Recognises past history of severe sinusitis

   Unsatisfactory   History achieves none of the above

2. **Information gathering – Physical examination**

   Good
   i) Views nose efficiently without causing discomfort
   ii) Views throat efficiently without causing gagging or discomfort
   iii) Checks for tenderness over the sinuses with gentle pressure

   Unsatisfactory   Candidate omits physical examination

3. **Doctor/Patient interaction – Patient's concerns**

   Good
   i) Sympathetic attitude, not dismissive of trivial condition, and identifies concern over special event before pt reveals it
   ii) Recognises expectation of antibiotics
   iii) Recognises concern that sinusitis could recur

   Unsatisfactory   Candidate ignores patient's concerns

4. **Communication – explanation**

   Good
   i) That this is chronic rhinitis
   ii) Likely to be caused by an allergy not bacteria
   iii) Antibiotics of no help in this situation

   Unsatisfactory   No explanation of condition

5. **Patient management – options**

   Good
   i) Option given between antihistamines v topical preparations
   ii) Pros and cons of above explained
   iii) Options of RAST testing or skin patch testing offered

   Unsatisfactory   None of these options offered

---

g – good   **s – satisfactory**   **b– barely adequate**   **n – not very good**
u – unsatisfactory   **o – omitted**

Seriously deficient performance

APPROACH TO MEMBERSHIP BY ASSESSMENT (MAP)

Most of us know GPs who take pride in providing a high quality service for their patients, but are not RCGP members. Although, for one reason or another they have not taken or passed the MRCGP exam, they support the aims of the college. Some are involved in postgraduate education, as GP trainers or GP tutors and some just want a more formal recognition of the quality of their service. They would like to join as full members of the college, but are daunted by the thought of sitting the exam.

The RCGP council agreed that, from 1999, experienced GPs could gain membership by a rigorous and reliable assessment of their day-to-day clinical work – including the necessary skills, practice organisation and continuing education. A wide variety of GPs from nine national GP bodies had chosen the aspects of a GP's work that should be assessed, in a process involving three stages. The method was developed and tested over the next year (Holden & Wearne in *Br J Gen Pract* March 2000 p231–5).

Members by assessment are not considered to be in any way different from those who have passed the exam. The assessment of the performance of clinical work by MAP may be considered a truer measure of quality than the exam, which measures competence – which is the ability to provide it.

What is the Standard?
MAP is based on the General Medical Council's *Good Medical Practice.* It assesses to a level of good but *real* General Practice – it is not a test of excellence – the college has different instruments to measure this. It should be equivalent to the level of care that could be provided by GPs who have maintained their standards since passing the MRCGP exam.

What does MAP Involve?
• Consultation Skills Assessment – Video or Simulated Surgery
Assessment of consultations is by the same method as for the exam. In fact, the Video and Simulated Surgery examiners are unaware which route the candidate is taking to membership. You must pass one of them before sending off the paperwork for the next stage. You can find further details in other chapters of this book.

- Written submission

The written submission includes ten sections that contain *essential* and *optional criteria*. You have to choose ten optional 'points' from the eighteen possible. See Appendices 1 and 2.

- Practice visit

These three sections can be submitted 'stepwise' or all together. Preparation of this material involves a significant amount of work, taking most busy GPs a year or two.

Written Submission Sections

1. Accessibility & continuity
2. Continuing professional development
3. Ethical standards
4. Health promotion
5. Management of acute illness
6. Management of chronic illness
7. Patient records
8. Practice organisation and team working
9. Prescribing and referral
10. Consultation

Written Evidence Types

- Practice procedures
- Clinical guidelines
- Practice statistics and audits
- Written work – reports on cases and education diaries

The type of evidence varies with the different criteria – from simple practice data, to office procedures and clinical guidelines (which should be in use), to specified logs of patients you have treated in different situations, and more detailed case reports. Several criteria require demonstration of a full audit cycle; this often takes the best part of a year. However you may be able to use one that you have already started – or even finished! Some criteria do specify how recently you must have collected the evidence – see Appendix 3.

When your written work has been assessed as satisfactory, the practice visit will be arranged. Two trained assessors, GPs practising away from your area, will visit your practice for the day. They will discuss your submission with you in a structured way and will also need to speak to your partners and other clinical and non-clinical members of your practice team. You should inform them that you are preparing for MAP at an early stage – and enlist their help wherever possible!

If the list seems rather daunting, remember that there are no tricks! You will only be assessed on the criteria described in the MAP Handbook. It has been written for the guidance of candidates and assessors. The whole process aims to be *transparent*. It should be unusual for a truthful candidate to fail at the stage of the visit. However, some may have given up after failing the consultation skills assessment, others during the preparation of the written submission.

All evidence you provide – video tape, written submission and during the practice visit – is treated in confidence, limited only by the GMC's *Duties of a Doctor*.

Steps in MAP Process

1. Contemplation
- Obtain a copy of the latest MAP Handbook – currently £10 from the MAP Administrator at the RCGP (020 7581 3232)
- Go to the website (www.rcgp.org.uk)
- Questions:
  Why do I want MRCGP?
  Do I have enough time at present? – How long will it take?
  How will I prepare? – Can I join a group?
  Why don't I just take the exam?
  Video or Simulated Surgery?

You should allow between one and three years for the whole process – one successful candidate logged 200 hours.

You may discover that there is a MAP preparation group nearby. When you apply, you will be offered a trained MAP adviser from your local RCGP faculty. You can probably get PGEA approval for your preparation – see your GP tutor. Your regional dean may be prepared to provide support if you are preparing to be a GP Trainer or Tutor. Check whether your Primary care organisation is running any initiatives that will help your preparation e.g. summarising notes, audits, patient questionnaires, in-practice education – you can suggest that they do!

The Simulated Surgery is expensive to run and costs significantly more (currently £225 extra). However, your video preparation will probably take at least two extra full days of your professional time. On the other hand, you have complete control of the material on which you will be assessed.

2. Application – Taking the plunge!
When you apply, you must have been in independent UK General Practice for five years and have worked in your current practice for at least three sessions a week for one year.

When should I apply?
You need to pull together a number of factors in this decision
* How long do I need for the preparation of my written submission?
* How long do I need to summarise 80% of my/our records?
* When can I get my CPR & CHS certificates?
* Do I have any existing work that will become 'out of date'? (Appendix 3)
* When will I be ready for the consultation skills assessment?
  The videos and Simulated Surgeries are only assessed twice a year, in May and December, with final application dates about three months before. Only limited numbers can be assessed each time, particularly for the Simulated Surgery. So you need to send your video tape, or book your Simulated Surgery slot as early as possible. You will only be sent the appropriate consultation skills workbook when your MAP application has been received.
* The MAP criteria are updated on 1st April each year (usually only slightly and to make them clearer)

You have three years from the time of your application to submit your written evidence. At this time, you will be able to choose whether it is assessed on the current criteria or those from the previous year.

Send a completed application form (from the handbook), the four certificates required and the administration fee. There are two further fees – you have to pay one when you send your video tape or book your Simulated Surgery place, the other when you send off your written submission.

Certificates Required on Application for MAP

1. GMC
2. RCGP Resuscitation Certificate – from the handbook
3. RCGP CHS Certificate – from the handbook or Health Authority confirmation on the CHS list
4. JCPTP or Health Authority Certificate confirming your eligibility as a GP in the UK

3. Consultation skills assessment

The Video and Simulated Surgery modules are described elsewhere in this book. You will receive a copy of a very informative workbook when you apply for MAP.

There is a common misconception that outcomes of the consultations are assessed – they are not, merely the presence of very clearly defined consulting skills (which usually together lead to a successful outcome).

The video has produced a significant hurdle for several MAP candidates. Although the video criteria were developed from the analysis of successful consultations involving experienced GPs, one consultation, even a very good one, rarely contains evidence that the GP has *all* the required skills. Just recording a surgery that seemed pretty good at the time is unlikely to produce the goods.

4. The written submission

It is beyond the scope of this chapter to explain all the criteria – they are clearly set out in the handbook. You can find a very abbreviated list in Appendix 1. It has been included to give you an idea of the sort of preparation necessary – please check the handbook carefully before starting any preparatory work. The RCGP is currently preparing a detailed *Users' Guide*.

MAP advisers and assessors agree that the most common problems arise from not reading the criteria carefully enough. You can find some of the more common 'mis-readings' in Appendix 4.

You can send off each of the ten sections separately and in any order – you must decide whether you want your whole submission to be assessed under the current or previous year's rules. You will get a reply within a few weeks: either that it has been accepted – or with guidance as to how your submission could be improved to reach the required standard. The whole process is meant to be educational – nearly all the successful MAP candidates have had to modify and resubmit some sections. Of course, this is less likely to happen if you let your MAP adviser see the work before you send it.

5. The practice visit

The trained assessors, two GPs you don't know, will visit your practice, on an agreed date – usually 2–6 months after all of your submission has been received.

They will have agreed a programme with you that may look something like this:

9.30	Meet candidate, introductions, brief tour of practice
9.50	1st interview with candidate
11.20	Assessors confer over coffee
11.40	Meet receptionists
12.15	Inspection of records, leaflets, referral letters
12.45	Appointment with another GP in the practice
13.00	Assessors confer over lunch
13.45	Appointment with Practice Manager
14.00	2nd interview with candidate
15.30	Assessors agree the report over tea
16.15–16.30	End

The assessors may want to clarify parts of your written submission. They will discuss your decision making in the various clinical situations you have presented. Remember – the assessors are working GPs like yourself, they have chosen the job because they believe in MAP and those who haven't passed the exam should have the opportunity to join the RCGP membership. They will try to encourage you and your team – but obviously they can't provide the answers to their questions. However, they will *only* be assessing you against the explicit criteria published in the handbook.

Functions of the practice visit
- Discuss your decision making
- Check your medical records, drugs, equipment, etc
- Check your contribution to the evidence
- Check your staff are using your procedures

If all goes well, they will recommend that you are admitted to membership of the RCGP, and you will receive a copy of their report within four weeks of the visit.

Other questions

What if it takes longer than I expected?

If you overrun the three years from application to submission of all of the written material, you can re-apply – it will cost you another administration fee. But remember:

Your video or Simulated Surgery pass only lasts three years

Some of your written work can become time expired (Appendix 3)

The three years may be extended in special circumstances (see the handbook).

Can non-principals take MAP?

As long as you have regularly worked three sessions a week in the practice for the year before you apply and continue to do so until the visit. It may be more difficult for you to influence some practice policies, but you will need to show that the care you provide is not compromised.

What if I am concerned that the care provided by my partner(s) will let me down?

The same applies, but it can be very difficult to be a good GP in a practice that is struggling. However, as MAP is a personal award your efforts will be recognised even if not successful across the whole practice.

My partner and I want to take MAP together – can we be visited together?

Yes, but for a maximum of two – the handbook provides details.

It seems a lot of work – are their any other benefits to MAP?

MAP should provide evidence for *Revalidation, Clinical Governance, Personal Learning Plans* and *Practice Professional Development Plans* – doubtless more will arrive over the next year or so.

Some GPs have decided to prepare for MAP when they realised that their Primary care organisation was using the RCGP Clinical Governance tool – *Quality Team Development* (*QTD*) – which shares several criteria with MAP. They have been able to use PCG/PCT support for this form of Clinical Governance to get them started.

Appendix 1: ABBREVIATED MAP

1. Accessibility and Continuity
a. Same day contact for urgent problems (log of 50 requests)
b. Emergency calls during surgery hours (practice procedure)
c. 7.5 min. average consultation (log of 50 consecutive consultations)
d. Routine appointment in 5 working days 1st available at start of 10 weeks
e. Continuity of care practice (policies and logs/surveys)

2. Continuing professional development/review of performance
abc 3 educational needs, how identified, met and evaluated
d. Report of 1 year's educational activity
e. Activity in up to three of:
Research-Investigation use; Skills development; EBM; Teaching
f. †Reflective diary for one month with some resulting changes
g. Significant event review – for 5 of a list of 10 suggestions

3. Ethical standards
a. Confidentiality policies, staff training & contract
b. Ethical dilemma description 200–800 words
c. Complaints procedure
d. Policies for non-discrimination patients, colleagues and staff
e. GMC certificate

4. Health promotion
a. Policy and audit for one area
b. for up to 3 more areas

5. Management of acute illness
a. Emergency drugs and equipment lists
b. CPR certificate
c. Competent decision-making log of 20 patients with acute illness
d. Emergency hospital admissions log of 5
e. †Out of Hours care log of 20 patients
f. †Information leaflets 10, with 3 patients' comments for each

6. Management of chronic illness
a. Clinical guidelines with justification, for 3 diseases from 10 listed
b. Audit cycles for the 3 i.e. 'before & after', in last year
c. †Diary of one terminal care patient
d. †Diary of one chronic debilitating illness patient
e. †Directory of 10 self-help groups with 5 recent examples of use

7. Patient records
a. Last entry in 20 random notes examined on the visit
b. Practice statistics age groups, turnover, 4 week's consultations
c. Age-sex distribution of patients with 3 chronic diseases in 6a
d. 80% records summarised paper, computer or a mix

8. Practice organisation and team working
a. Urgent and routine access for telephone messages, letters, etc
b. PCHT contact arrangements 6 groups listed
c. 3 case reports of PCHT communication
d. Practice leaflet
e. †Practice team learning programme for 6m in last 2 years
f. †Practice development report significant change in last 2 years

9. Prescribing and referral
a. Prescribing review one group of drugs, over 3m in last 2 years
b. Repeat prescribing system log of 100 consecutive repeats
c. Generic prescribing rate e.g. PACT report
d. Referral letters all in previous 6m
e. Evaluation of 10 referrals up to 300 words total – 1° and 2° care
f. Directory of local services

10. Consultation
a. Consulting skills assessment already passed by this stage
b. †Analysis of 50 patient satisfaction survey

† = optional criteria points – choose 10 from 18

NB Please refer to the handbook for definitive criteria descriptions

Appendix 2: 'OPTIONAL' MAP CRITERIA 2001

NB You must choose ten points – or – omit only eight!

Continuing Professional Development/Review of performance

2e	Demonstrate activity in up to three of:	**up to 3 points**
	• Research	
	• Investigation review	
	• Skills development	
	• Evidence-based medicine	
	• Contribution to medical education	
2f	1 month Reflective diary	**1 point**
2g	10 Significant event reviews	**3 points**

Health Promotion

4b	3 extra health promotion audits	**up to 3 points**

Management of acute illness

5e	Out of hours survey – 20 patients	**1 point**
5f	10 acute illness leaflets – 3 patients' comments for each	**1 point**

Management of chronic illness

6c	Terminal care report	**1 point**
6d	Chronic debilitating illness report	**1 point**
6e	10 self-help/support agencies – 5 reports of use	**1 point**

Practice organisation and team working

8e	Report of 6m Practice Team continuing professional development programme	**1 point**
8f	Report of involvement in practice's development for 2 years	**1 point**

Consultation

10b	Analysis of survey of 50 patients' satisfaction with their consultations	**1 point**

Appendix 3: TIME LIMITATIONS on 2001 MAP CRITERIA

NB Other criteria may be discussed on the visit – easier with recent cases

1. Accessibility and continuity

a	Log of 50 consecutive requests for urgent consultations	**in last year**
b	Log of 50 consecutive consultations	**in last year**
c	Log of 1st routine appt. at start of 10 consecutive weeks	**in last year**
e	Continuity of care surveys – out of hours communication, palliative care, follow-up visits & surgery consultations	**in last year**

2. Continuing professional development/review of performance

abc	Descriptions of identifying, meeting & evaluating 3 substantial educational needs	**in last 5 years**
d	Description of educational activities	**in last year**

5. Management of acute illness

b	Resuscitation Certificate (submit on application) (same for Child Health Surveillance Certificate)	**in last 3 years**

6. Management of chronic illness

a	3 Chronic illness management plans	**published/updated in last 3 years**
b	Double audits of aspects of 6a within 1 year	**completed in last year**
c	Terminal care report	**died in last year <u>or</u> terminally ill for 3m**

7. Patient records

b	Practice turnover statistics for 12 months	**'recent'**
c	Candidate's consultation statistics for 4 weeks	**'recent'**

8. Practice organisation and team working

d	Practice Leaflet	**in last year**
e	Report of 6m Practice Team continuing professional development programme	**in last 2 years**
f	Report of involvement in practice's development	**in last 2 years**

9. Prescribing and referral

c	Prescription survey	**in last year**
d	Copies of all referral letters	**in last 6 months**

Appendix 4: TIPS FOR SOME CRITERIA

1.

b (ii) A list of emergency symptoms for the staff – NHS Direct or the ambulance service may be able to help

c 7.5 minute **face to face** patient contact in consultations – exclude time between patients e.g. for writing notes or telephone calls

2.

abc Ask your GP tutor for help with these *Personal Learning Plans*

a A description of **how & why** the educational need was discovered – it's not enough to say: I realised it while attending the lecture that then met the need. Evidence within the *Reflective Diary* (2f) or *Significant Event Reviews* (2g) may also be used for this.

b Remember to justify your choice of learning method

e **Personal** research – you should have had an important role in its design and writing the report.
Personal outcomes from local or regional GP Trainer or Tutor workshops can be described.

f The diary should reveal that **some** of the reflection has resulted in action e.g. personal learning, practice policy – not just comments on the vagaries of General Practice, etc.

g These reviews should include formal **discussions** with colleagues

3.

b The ethical dilemma description should include stating the pros & cons for a difficult decision, with a justification for your choice.

4.

ab Justify the local relevance, and evidence base for the activity.

5.

a Make sure your emergency drugs are in date & that there are maintenance arrangements for your equipment.

cde You have chosen these 20 + 5 + 20 patients – discuss your management decisions with colleagues before the assessor's visit

f   Consider handing out a short patient feedback questionnaire with the leaflets

6.

a   Your 3 practice chronic disease management plans should be less than 3yrs old and based on national or local referenced guidelines.

b   This 'double' audit will often take a year – start early & don't try to audit every aspect of your management plans. The print-outs from most GP systems are not very neat – but they can be tidied.

cd   Remember to describe how you involved **others** in the team

8.

c   Include your **reasons** for, & the **content** of the communication

f   Yours should have been a major part in this practice development

Appendix 5

VIDEO SCORE SHEET (<u>before</u> viewing)

1 column for each consultation – tick the skills you think you've shown

Consultation Description and age/sex										
Start time										
Why patient came	~	~	~	~	~	~	~	~	~	~
Encourages patient's contribution										
Responds to cues										
Gets psycho-social context										
	~	~	~	~	~	~	~	~	~	~
Define the problem	~	~	~	~	~	~	~	~	~	~
Doesn't miss serious condition										
Chooses examination										
Makes working diagnosis										
	~	~	~	~	~	~	~	~	~	~
Explain	~	~	~	~	~	~	~	~	~	~
Explains diag, mgt & treatment										
Appropriate language										
	~	~	~	~	~	~	~	~	~	~
Addresses problem	~	~	~	~	~	~	~	~	~	~
Appropriate management plan										
Shares management options										
	~	~	~	~	~	~	~	~	~	~
Effective consulting	~	~	~	~	~	~	~	~	~	~
Appropriate prescribing or not										
Rapport										

SUMMATIVE ASSESSMENT

The NHS (Vocational Training for General Medical Practice) Regulations 1997 made the passing of Summative Assessment mandatory by law for all GP Registrars who started their 12 months as a GP registrar after 30 January 1998. The Joint Committee on Postgraduate Training for General Practice (JCPTGP) and Directors of Postgraduate General Practice Education are committed to Summative Assessment as a test of GP Registrars' skills, ensuring that those completing training achieve a minimum level of competence to practise independently as General Practitioners.

A National Summative Assessment Board is responsible for administering, monitoring and, in some cases, organising, the components of Summative Assessment approved by the JCPTGP, in the Deaneries. It operates on behalf of the Conference of General Practice Education Directors (COGPED). At a local level the Deanery Office is responsible for administration and all enquiries should be addressed there.

Currently there is a major review of the organisation of licensing requirements and changes may be introduced.

Why is summative assessment necessary?
There are a number of reasons why Summative Assessment has been introduced. The following are of particular importance:

- To assess competence
- To reassure the public and protect patients from doctors whose performance is not adequate
- To reassure individual doctors that they have achieved a minimum standard of competence
- To identify those who are not ready for independent practice and require further training or who may need to reconsider their career options

What are the basic attributes tested by summative assessment?
- Knowledge
- Problem solving skills
- Clinical competence
- Consulting/communication skills
- Skills in producing a written report of practical work in General Practice
- Performance on a wide variety of skills, attitudes and knowledge, confirmed by a structured trainer's report

What are the components of summative assessment?
There are four components which cover the six basic attributes. In three of the component areas candidates have a choice of the method by which they will be tested (Table 1). In order to receive a certificate of prescribed/equivalent experience (without which you cannot practice as a GP, locum or deputy) it is necessary to pass all four parts.

Table 1: Components and approved methods of Summative Assessment

1.	**MULTIPLE CHOICE QUESTIONNAIRE (MCQ)**
➤	The COGPED MCQ or
➤	The MRCGP MCQ examination
2.	**ASSESSMENT OF CONSULTING SKILLS**
➤	The COGPED Video Component or
➤	The MRCGP Assessment of Consulting Skills (Video) Module or
➤	The Leicester/Yorkshire Simulated Patient Surgery
3.	**WRITTEN SUBMISSION OF PRACTICAL WORK**
➤	The COGPED Audit or
➤	The National Project Marking Schedule
4.	**STRUCTURED TRAINER'S REPORT**

Multiple Choice Questionnaire (MCQ)
The COGPED MCQ paper lasts three hours, tests knowledge and problem-solving skills, and is held on four separate occasions each year. Deanery Offices publish local venues and dates. It is unwise to undertake the MCQ before completing at least three months of General Practice-based training because the paper contains specific General Practice elements.

Questions cover all areas found in General Practice. The proportion of questions in each area is as follows:

- Internal medicine (medicine, therapeutics, surgical diagnosis, psychiatry, geriatrics, etc.) – 45% of total
- Child health – one sixth of the total
- Women's health – one sixth of the total
- External medicine (ENT, eyes, dermatology) – one sixth of the total
- Practice management – 5% of total

The paper consists currently of two types of question, true/false questions and extended matching questions. The proportion of each may vary but there are currently 260 of the former and 40 of the latter variety. Similar questions are used in the MRCGP MCQ and examples of such questions can be found in that section of this book.

GP Registrars who fail can resit at the next available opportunity. However issues surrounding failure should be discussed with Trainer, Course Organiser or Associate Director. A registrar who starts the year in August can have three attempts within that year (December, February and May) before having to apply for extended training as a consequence of failing. There is no charge to take the COGPED MCQ.

The pass mark at each sitting varies according to the difficulty of the paper. It is determined by a group of examiners estimating the expected performance of a notional GP Registrar of minimum acceptable competence. The pass rate is approximately 94% at each sitting.

Most candidates will have the required level of knowledge from medical school and hospital experience. However it is advisable to practice MCQ papers beforehand. From these it should be easy to identify gaps in knowledge and direct reading accordingly.

GP Registrars who pass the MCQ module of the MRCGP examination, will receive a letter from the College to this effect. This can be used as an alternative to the COGPED MCQ as evidence of adequate performance in this component of Summative Assessment.

Assessment of consulting skills
The majority of candidates use a video for this part of the assessment. They have one of two options. They may submit a video to the Deanery Office for assessment by COGPED examiners. Alternatively a pass achieved in this module of the MRCGP examination will also be accepted as evidence of competence in consulting skills for Summative Assessment. Should a pass in the latter not be obtained the video tape will be 'fast tracked' and automatically enter the COGPED Summative Assessment process. This process is known as the MRCGP/SA single route video.

Video tapes that fail MRCGP may still pass the COGPED Summative Assessment process. MRCGP requires a relative consistency of performance across specific criteria and some failing candidates may fall short in one or two areas only but otherwise show reasonable consulting skills. The COGPED process relies less on counting the number of times specific criteria have been demonstrated and makes a more global assessment of performance.

The National Summative Assessment Board has published a list of required skills for success in the COGPED process (Table 2). In reality the best way to be sure of adequate performance is to demonstrate the MRCGP criteria irrespective of the chosen route. For instance identifying the reason for a patient's attendance requires encouragement of the patient's contribution, responses to relevant cues, identification of psychological or social factors and consideration of the patient's agenda/health understanding. Reaching an agreement with the patient requires explanation of diagnosis and negotiation of treatment. All these are MRCGP criteria. Candidates who submit a lower standard of video for the COGPED process risk failure.

Table 2: Skills required in COGPED video process

• Identify the reasons for the patient's attendance
• Take appropriate steps to investigate the problems presented
• Organise a suitable management plan
• Reach an agreement with the patient on diagnosis and treatment
• Demonstrate an understanding (in the logbook) of what was going on in the consultation

The acquisition of competent consulting skills is probably the most important element in the transition from Registrar to GP. To consult in a satisfactory manner requires a patient-centred approach. Using techniques such as open questions, silence and echoing, followed by the skilful use of relevant direct questions, will encourage the maximum contribution from the patient.

Consultations are still submitted in which no attempt has been made to elicit the patient's agenda (i.e. their ideas, concerns and expectations) and if this is persistent throughout the tape, the candidate will fail. It may be necessary to ask direct questions to reach it. However once the patient's agenda is clear the exploration of psychological factors becomes easier. This is something that Registrars often find difficult particularly when faced with an apparent physical problem. It is also advisable to include some consultations in which patients present directly with psychological problems. Such patients will also more readily divulge information about the social background to their problem, making the Registrar's task easier.

Examiners are looking for candidates to demonstrate quite a high level of proficiency in consulting skills. Emphasis is on the word demonstrate. This, after all, is an examination. In a normal surgery there will be many consultations in which a doctor will not need to use the full range of skills. These low challenge consultations should not be submitted for Summative Assessment because skills cannot be adequately demonstrated. Patients presenting with new problems are the best. Follow-up consultations are more difficult, as are consultations where a diagnosis is not necessary such as when issuing a certificate or repeat prescription. If there is only one sensible line of management it is not easy to share management options. Difficult problems may be daunting but they are good for demonstrating skills.

The COGPED process does not only look at consulting skills. It also looks for clinical competence. Minor errors, unless they occur frequently, may be overlooked. A major error that could potentially harm the patient will stop a pass at the first level and result in referral to second-level examiners. Ignoring cues suggestive of a serious physical or psychological problem would be regarded as a major error. So too would be a failure to check for suicide risk in a patient who is significantly depressed.

A logbook is submitted with the video. In this the Registrar has to demonstrate they understand the process and outcome of the consultation. This is an opportunity to highlight skills displayed. Background information, for instance social context, can be mentioned in the logbook but it is better for this to come out in the consultation. Examiners pay most attention to what they see, and an outline of the patient's concerns in the logbook will not make up for failure to elicit them on video. Shortcomings should also be noted but, if these are too obvious, it is better not to submit that consultation in the first place.

The regulations and technical details about video recording should be obtained from the Deanery Office for the COGPED Summative Assessment process and from the RCGP about the MRCGP/SA Single Route Video. Blank tapes are provided by the Deanery. A two-hour recording should be submitted. The average length of consultations should be no greater than 15 minutes. This should result in a minimum of eight consultations on the tape but as more are expected in the COGPED process some shorter consultations are required. In the

MRCGP/SA route the first five consultations on the tape will be examined for the MRCGP. If a consultation lasts longer than 15 minutes the examiner may not watch the excess time.

In its guidance to candidates the National Summative Assessment Board suggests that taping of an ordinary surgery throughout is usually adequate and it should not be necessary to spend large amounts of time editing the video tape. This displays some optimism on their part that every consultation will be suitable for the adequate demonstration of skills. It is certainly too optimistic if the MRCGP/SA route is being followed. There the first five consultations should represent a 'masterpiece'.

It is important to begin regular video recordings early in the registrar year and look at these with the trainer. Early efforts may look awkward, but continued practice will be rewarded. It may help to keep a list of the MRCGP criteria on the desk for easy reference. More difficult criteria can be practised in turn. When consultations appear to be of the right standard it will be helpful for the trainer or course organiser to comment. The final choice of consultations should rest with the candidate. The key points for success are summarised in Table 3.

Table 3: Summative Assessment video, key points for success.

• Start recording early and record regularly
• Practise more difficult skills in turn
• Check the patient's ideas, concerns and expectations
• Explain the diagnosis and negotiate management with the patient
• Exclude consultations in which there are clinical errors
• Demonstrate skills on the video, rather than recording what might have happened in the logbook

Videos must be presented no later than three months before the end of the General Practice training. In the COGPED process two first level examiners view the recording. If both are satisfied the candidate passes. If either is not satisfied the tape is referred to a second level at which a decision to pass or refer to national level is made. The final decision is taken at national level. In the event of failure it is normal to apply for an extension of training.

An alternative to the video is a Simulated Patient Surgery. This was pioneered by the Yorkshire and South Trent Deaneries and is available to all GP registrars in the UK, with the permission of their Regional Director. Various centres within these two Deaneries are used for the test and either Deanery Office can be contacted for details. Yorkshire is usually used for northern applicants and South Trent for southern applicants. Candidates should attempt the Simulated Patient Surgery during the second six months of training in General Practice. A candidate sees eight patient simulators during the surgery and the consultations last ten minutes each. Following each consultation the simulator completes a patient satisfaction sheet and a clinical checklist. Those who fail to demonstrate adequate consulting skills in at least six of the eight consultations are required to carry out a further eight consultation surgeries in which five consultations must be passed. If a pass is not achieved on the second surgery an expert panel takes the final pass-fail decision.

Written submission of practical work
The written submission of practical work can be:

- an audit as organised by the COGPED
- a project marked under the National Project Marking Schedule

The written submission can be completed at any time during the three years of vocational training but submitted no later than three months before the end of the General Practice year. The work must be relevant to General Practice. It is to the GP Registrar's advantage to submit the work as early as possible in case resubmission becomes necessary.

Audit has been chosen because all General Practitioners should monitor and improve the quality of care they provide. These skills form a key part of clinical governance within primary care. The ability to carry out an audit is therefore a skill of minimal competence for a GP registrar. The audit should be the GP registrar's own work with appropriate support from the practice team. An eight criteria complete audit cycle has been introduced to replace the old seven criteria method in which the cycle was not completed (Table 4). In order to pass all criteria must be present.

Table 4: Eight Criterion Audit Cycle

Reason for choice of audit	The subject area should be relevant to the practice and have potential for change
Criterion/Criteria chosen	Criteria should be important to the study area and justifiable e.g. by reference to literature
Standards set	Reasons should be given for the choice of standards e.g. local advice or literature
Preparation and planning	Outline the preparation for data collection and difficulties encountered with evidence of teamwork and discussion where appropriate
Data collection (1)	Present results in a suitable form and compare them against the standard. Data should permit appropriate conclusions to be drawn
Change(s) to be evaluated	What changes are being implemented? How were they decided and why?
Data collection (2)	Compare the results with data collection (1) and the standards
Conclusions	Summarise what has been learnt from the audit

The best advice about the audit is to keep it simple and relevant. It should be related to an activity that has direct bearing on a GP registrar's work, ideally where change is desired or expected. It helps if there is adequate literature on the topic. The five most popular audit topics from one Deanery show that many GP registrars already follow this advice (Table 5). The work should not exceed 3000 words. If the assessors are not satisfied the audit will be returned for further work. Advice should be sought from the GP trainer, Course Organiser and/or Deanery Co-ordinator before attempting modifications and resubmission. Only then if it remains unsatisfactory will it fail.

Table 5: Most popular audit topics, North West England Deanery

- Is the management of hypertension in diabetic patients adequate?
- Are patients on ACE inhibitors having their urea and electrolytes checked?
- Are lipid levels in patients with ischaemic heart disease managed appropriately?
- Is the monitoring of patients taking thyroxine replacement adequate?
- Are patients taking long-term corticosteroids receiving treatment to prevent osteoporosis?

The National Project Marking Schedule has been introduced to widen the choice of written submission options. It is available to all GP Registrars in the UK through the Yorkshire Deanery and some other Deaneries. If it is not offered locally, submissions may be sent to Yorkshire with the signed consent of the local director. The available options are shown in Table 6.

Table 6: Options available under the National Project Marking Schedule

- Questionnaire study
- Review of notes
- Literature review
- Clinical case study (or case series)
- Research study
- Plan for a new service in the practice
- Audit
- Discussion paper

Detailed guidelines have been produced for candidates on how to structure the project. They can be obtained form the local Deanery or the Yorkshire Deanery. Before preparing a project, GP registrars are strongly advised to read these and to follow them carefully while carrying out and writing up the project. From the point of view of marking the project is divided into six areas and candidates must pass each area. Details are shown in Table 7.

The choice of project options allows scope for innovation. The National Project Marking Schedule is designed to mark high quality projects as well as those of minimum acceptable standard. The former will be given higher marks as distinct from the simple pass/fail of the other components of Summative Assessment. As with audit, if assessors are not satisfied with the project it will be returned for further work.

Table 7: Project structure

1.	Statement of aims	There should be a clear statement of one or more of aims, objectives, question, hypothesis, problem and reason for the study. Better candidates will develop arguments, derive aims from them and show the relevance of the study to practice.
2.	Reference to literature	Normally six or more relevant references will be listed at the end and referred to clearly in the text. Ideally literature should be used to develop arguments and derive reasons for the project.
3.	Method clearly stated	It should be appropriate, practical and ethical so that a reader could repeat it. Higher marks are given for good design, piloting, reasons for method and quality of analysis of findings.
4.	Presentation of evidence	Relate evidence to aims and present it clearly. Use different ways to show numerical data. An explanation of missing data, a presentation that reflects arguments and overall elegance of style will secure high marks.
5.	Discussion of evidence	How well has the method addressed the aims? Are the findings relevant to the practice and likely to bring about change? To score highly consider how change may be effected and its implications. Compare with other work.
6.	Conclusions	Evidence presented should justify the conclusions. Better candidates will make suggestions for improvement and look at the need for further work.

Structured trainer's report

This is a document in which evidence of the GP registrar's performance is collected and recorded. For each item of the report, the trainer should document sufficient information to enable him/her to make a judgment as to whether the GP Registrar has achieved the standard for independent practice. Thirty-one items make up the report (Table 8) and GP Registrars have to reach a satisfactory standard in each.

Table 8: Components of the Structured Trainer's Report

Main Headings	Section Headings	Items (Titles abbreviated)
Part 1 Specific Clinical Skills	**Specific Clinical Skills**	1. Mental State 2. Using the Auriscope 3. Using the Ophthalmoscope 4. Using the Sphygmomanometer 5. Using the Stethoscope 6. Using the Peak Flow Meter 7. The Vaginal Examination 8. Using the Vaginal Speculum 9. The Cervical Smear 10. The Rectal Examination 11. Venous Access 12. I.M. and S.C Injection
Part 2 Patient Care **Management**	**Making a Diagnosis**	13. Communication skills 14. Recognise common physical, psychological problems 15. Includes ideas, concerns, expectations 16. Knowledge and skills to deal with life events 17. Examines each system and organ proficiently 18. Examines with appropriate consideration
	Patient	19. The doctor chooses appropriate management 20. Broad knowledge of all aspects of drugs 21. Diagnosis and manages acute emergencies 22. Appropriate care and support for patients and families
	Clinical Judgment	23. Undertakes appropriate examination 24. Responds to requests for urgent attendance
Part 3 Personal Skills	**Organisation Skills**	25. Aware of own limitations 26. The doctor is able to manage their own time 27. Understands the obligations of a GP
	Professional Values	28. Possesses and applies ethical principles 29. Maintains own physical and mental health 30. Accepts appropriate responsibility
	Personal and Professional Growth	31. The doctor is able to identify strengths and weakness in his/her performance

The final decision about standards rests with the trainer. Evidence must be presented to support that decision. This can come from a variety of sources and will vary according to each item in the report. The trainer can seek advice from others when necessary. Each item is listed separately in the report and in order to assist the trainer, fail criteria and sources of evidence have been added (Table 9)

Table 9: One Item from the Structured Trainer's Report

16	*The Doctor has the knowledge and skills to deal with life events and crises.*	Evidence collection complete

Fail Criteria

The Doctor repeatedly fails to:

- Recognise or understand the importance of life events and crises to patients.
- Respond to life events or crises presented to him/her.
- Utilise the resources available to deal with such events (including material, personal or professional resources).

Methods	Date	Comments
❑ Observations		
❑ Video		
❑ Case analysis		
❑ Simulated patient		
❑ Other		

GP Registrars should discuss the Structured Trainer's Report with their GP trainer early in their training to ensure that they are familiar with the relevant areas of practice. They can also assist in its completion by drawing the trainer's attention when a particular procedure is being carried out. Trainers find most difficulty in observing the simpler clinical skills and management of emergencies. In this context it is acceptable for the trainer to refer to a Registrar's hospital logbook for evidence provided they are sure that the evidence is reliable.

If a Registrar works closely with the trainer it should be easy to see any areas of difficulty and take steps to improve. It is persistent poor performance that causes failure. We are all allowed to make mistakes, although of course the seriousness of the mistake must be taken into consideration. The final decision is taken after 11 months of training in General Practice. If the year is split between two trainers the second trainer makes the final judgement. The first trainer contributes to this decision and fills in any sections of the report that he/she feels able to.

Applying for extended training

If a Registrar fails Summative Assessment and after discussion with the trainer, course organiser and associate director decides that he/she still wants to pursue a career in General Practice then further training must be applied for. Most Registrars only fail one component, usually the video, and show reasonable competence in other areas. It is usual to apply to the JCPTGP for a period of six months' extended training. It is not advisable to apply for less because there is one opportunity to apply.

Some doctors will need all this time to bring their skills up to the required standards. Others will not find it difficult and may feel that they have been unlucky in the original assessment. They should regard the extra time as an opportunity to learn more about General Practice. Those few schemes that offer more than the standard three years of training from the outset are usually highly sought after.

MRCGP – A REGISTRAR'S VIEW

Dr Louise R Newson

Preparation for the MRCGP exam is not easy! I found it quite a challenge entering general practice after five years of hospital medicine. Initially, the amount of information needed to pass the exam and, perhaps more importantly, to become a GP seemed completely overwhelming and daunting. It became rapidly apparent that GPs need to be 'jacks of all trades' rather then the 'master of one' that many hospital consultants I have worked for strived to be.

Looking back at the year, I think it is invaluable not to panic – after all, it should be an enjoyable year! My trainer was excellent at setting the pace and not pressurising me too much at the start. The beginning of the year was an important time to settle into the completely new working environment which was certainly a marked contrast to any I had experienced in hospitals.

Much of the exam still focuses on non-clinical information and I spent some time with different primary care members at the beginning of the year, which was actually very enlightening an educational. In retrospect it was far easier trying to understand various roles form the outset rather then finding yourself at the end of the year wondering who actually does the over 75 health checks, how temporary residents are claimed for, who deals with complaints in the practice or how receptionists spend their time in between surgeries!

At the start of the year I listed my 'areas of weakness' – this certainly was not difficult to do! I arranged to sit in at some local specialist out-patient clinics in some of these areas, eg ENT, Ophthalmology and Dermatology. It was far easier to organise this at the start of the year as my surgeries were easier to cancel than later on when patients were already booked in to see me.

Working through the PEP 2000 CD-Roms and several MCQ books was another useful way of finding out my weaker areas of knowledge. It was all too easy and tempting to stick to areas I felt comfortable with for topics for my tutorials – my trainer soon saw straight through me! The object of the tutorials is to learn and feel ignorant I suppose!

The amount of teaching / tutorials from trainers varied enormously in our local VTS group – from sporadic, rushed 'ad hoc' tutorials in coffee breaks to weekly 3 hour tutorials with an organised timetable. Longer tutorials are not necessarily better ones – so much really seems to depend upon the registrars' and trainers' personalities and also the learning needs and capabilities of the registrars.

My weekly tutorials were at a planned time but were not structured – they were usually discussions of problem patients or current management issues within the practice. Sometimes they evolved to conversations about politics, interesting novels and current films worth seeing; which, at the time, seemed like a complete waste of time, but by the time the oral exam came around I could understand their value and relevance!

My trainer was annoyingly good at questioning me, which I found completely frustrating at times. For an example, I would begin a tutorial by asking 'what would be the best way of managing a child with a UTI?'. The reply would be: 'What did you do?' Then: 'What do you know about childhood UTIs? Yes, but what else? And what else? Mmm, you must know more than that! Well, how are you going to find out more? What would you type into Medline? What would you expect to learn from this?' And so the questions continued!

The value of these exercises (fruitless as they seemed at the time) was actually immense. This 'questioning' approach has given me an excellent foundation and also new skills for dealing with general practice. Questioning everything I do during my working day certainly creates far too many questions to all be answered, but it also means that I can maintain my curiosity and my thirst for more knowledge.

I have also found questioning a very useful tool to use after consultations. For examples: Why did I do/say that? What could I have done differently? Did the patient leave my room satisfied? What have I learnt from this? This is all part of reflective learning, which really is the best and most effective method of learning for the exam and also for answering questions in the exam

Although I did not start to revise for the written exam until about two months before the exam, my trainer made me video some of my consultations from the first month of being a registrar. This was extremely useful, as it took at least three weeks for me work out the optimal position to place the camera for both myself and the patient to be in view and also to work out all the technicalities of the equipment (which, like many of my friends' cameras, was very temperamental)! We spent a lot of time watching my consultations on tape which I thought then was a complete waste of time. Once I had recovered from facing up to reality that I needed a new haircut and complete makeover to look half-way decent on film, I learnt so much from the earlier consultations. I was often surprised to see I really was not picking up on any cues at all from patients or even listening to them properly – I just seemed to have my own agenda and list of medical questions to work through for each new problem presented.

I had a regular surgery time for videoing, which worked really well – this was a late morning surgery so I was the only doctor consulting at that time. This meant the receptionists had time to give out the consent forms and explanations to the patients. I also had 15 minute consultations throughout the year for this surgery – which I needed to sort myself out in-between patients!

Although I started videoing so early on in the year, I found the videos by far the hardest and most time-consuming part of the exam. Objectively, it seems quite straight-forward when I read the guidelines from the college and saw the criteria to fulfil, but subjectively I felt it was an impossible task!

Having the list of criteria written out on a piece of card (away from the view of the camera!) was useful to refer to during consultations. Sharing management options was certainly the hardest part to do well (and the part most people fail on) so I spent a vast amount of time talking about different treatment options and really trying to put the ball in the patient's court when making a decision.

I went on a revision course at the end of January which was an ideal time, as it meant there was a lot of time to plan a revision schedule before the exam in May. It also meant that we were not too stressed at failing the pre-course exams!

Most of our VTS group divided ourselves into small groups of 4–5 people following this course. We tried to meet every week to go through old questions and also some 'Hot Topics'. This was useful, as often people had thought of completely different points of view about the same question.

'Hot Topics' was a very difficult area to revise as the amount of information needed to assimilate in a very short space of time appeared colossal. Many of us spent hours summarising the main journals, which really transpired to be quite a waste of time. It is probably more valuable to go on a 'Hot Topics' course and/or buy a 'Hot Topics' book.

Practising mock (or old) exam questions within the time constraints given for the exam is essential. The time allowed for Paper 2 is very generous. However, although 3½ hours seems a very long time, it flies by at a rate of knots during the exam. It is worthwhile trying to judge how long it takes to answer most standard questions and also having a framework for setting out the answers and some useful key phrases can be very useful.

The 'build-up' for the exam day can be very tiring. Creating the final recording for the video tape and completing the log book took me far longer than I had envisaged. This combined with last minute revision (or cramming) means it can be very tempting to have a few late nights and stressful days in the week or so preceding the exam.

However, it can not be overstated enough that the exam day is incredibly tiring. As many of the questions need logical common sense answers rather than high-flying facts, it really does pay off not to be exhausted on the day. The oral exam is another time when it is useful not to turn up to completely shattered.

Overall, it was a real relief to complete (and pass!) the exam during my registrar year. The MRCGP is a very relevant and fair exam and I found it a bonus to realise that most of my revision was not wasted knowledge as it is all used for everyday general practice.

APPENDIX 1: THE CONSULTATION

Various models have been described to help explain what happens in a consultation. The following summary of the various approaches is given to allow an overall view of the subject.

Description of events occurring in a consultation (after Byrne and Long 1976)

This model was produced after analysing over 2,000 tape recordings of consultations. They identified six phases that form a logical structure to the consultation.

- The doctor establishes a relationship with the patient.
- The doctor either attempts to discover, or actually discovers, the reason for the patient's attendance.
- The doctor conducts a verbal or physical examination, or both.
- The doctor, or the doctor and the patient together, or the patient alone (usually in that order of probability) consider(s) the condition.
- The doctor, and occasionally the patient, details treatment or further investigation.
- The consultation is terminated – usually by the doctor.

Expansion to include preventative care

In 1979 Stott and Davies described four areas which could be systematically explored each time a patient consults:

- Management of presenting problems
- Management of continuing problems
- Modification of help-seeking behaviour
- Opportunistic health promotion

A Model of Seven Tasks

This model was detailed by Pendleton *et al* in 1984. It lists seven tasks which form an effective consultation. The model emphasises the importance of the patient's view and understanding of the problem.

- To define the reasons for the patient's attendance including:
  The nature and history of the problem
  The cause of the problem

The patient's ideas, concerns and expectations
The effects of the problems
- To consider other problems:
Continuing problems
Risk factors
- To choose with the patient an appropriate action for each problem.
- To achieve a shared understanding with the patient.
- To involve the patient in the management plan and encourage him/her to accept appropriate responsibility.
- To use time and resources appropriately.
- To establish or maintain a relationship with the patient which helps to achieve the other tasks.

Health Belief Model

This model was devised by Rosenstock in 1966, and Becker and Maiman in 1975. It looks at the patient's reasons for accepting or rejecting the doctor's opinion. It shows that the patient is more likely to accept advice, diagnosis or treatment if the doctor is aware of their ideas, concerns and expectations.

It looks at various factors:

- Patient's interest in health varies – 'health motivation'.
- Patients vary in how likely they think they are to contract an illness – 'perceived vulnerability'.
- Patient's belief in the diagnosis is affected by whether they feel their opinion or 'concerns' have been understood by the doctor.
- 'Perceived seriousness' varies between patients for a given condition.

Six categories of intervention

This was devised by a psychologist, John Heron, in the mid-1970s, as a model of interventions which can be used by the doctor.

- Prescriptive: Instructions or advice – directive.
- Informative: Explaining and giving information.
- Confronting: Giving feedback to the patient on their behaviour or attitude, in order to help them see what is happening.
- Cathartic: Helping the patient to release their emotions.

- Catalytic: Encouraging the patient to explore their own feelings and reasons for their behaviour.
- Supportive: Encouraging the patient's self-worth e.g. by giving approval.

Transactional Analysis

This model of communication was described by Eric Berne in the 1960s. It explores our behaviour within relationships. It identifies three 'ego-states', parent, adult and child, any one of which an individual could be experiencing at any time. It looks at the implications and reasons for the different states. It also explores 'games', which can be used to identify why transactions repeatedly go wrong.

This model is useful for exploring consultations by looking at the relationship between the doctor and the patient.

Balint

This work in the 1950s explored the importance of the doctor–patient relationship. It explored the importance and identification of psychological problems. It suggested the following concepts:
- The doctor as the drug.
  The 'pharmacology' of the doctor as a treatment.
- The child as the presenting complaint.
  The patient may offer another person as the problem when there are underlying psycho-social problems.
- Elimination by appropriate physical examination.
  This may reinforce the patient's belief that their symptoms (neurotic in origin) are in fact due to physical illness. Repeated investigations perpetuate this cycle.
- Collusion of anonymity.
  As above, referral reinforces mistaken belief in the origin of symptoms. The responsibility of uncovering underlying psycho-social problems becomes increasingly diluted by repeated referral, with nobody taking final responsibility.
- The Mutual Investment Company.
  This is formed and managed by the doctor and the patient. 'Clinical illnesses' are episodes in a long relationship and represent 'offers' of problems (physical and psycho-social) to the doctor.

- The flash.
  The point in the consultation when the real reason of the 'offer' (underlying psycho-social and neurotic illness) is suddenly apparent to both doctor and patient. This forms a fulcrum for change; the consultation can now deal with the underlying basic 'fault'.

The Inner Consultation

This work by Roger Neighbour published in 1987 looks at improving consultation skills. He uses the following format for the consultation:

- Connecting: Rapport building skills
- Summarising: Listening and eliciting skills
- Handover: Communicating skills
- Safety netting: Predicting skills. Contingency plans of what and when further action may be needed.
- Housekeeping: Taking care of yourself, checking you are ready for the next patient.

It is not suggested that you should memorise the above models, but you should have an understanding of at least some of them. You should also be aware of how you can analyse your own consultation methods and how you could work on improving them i.e. use of video or audio tape recordings, simulated consultations with actors, role play or colleagues 'sitting in'.

APPENDIX 2: MEDICAL AUDIT

This has been defined as *'the systematic critical analysis of the quality of medical care, including the procedures used for diagnosis and treatment, the use of resources and the resulting outcome and quality of care of life for the patient.'* Department of Health, January 1989. A knowledge of the basic principles is essential, not just for the exam but also for day-to-day practice.

Medical audit can be seen as a series of steps (The Audit Cycle):

- Step 1   Choose a topic and set a standard
- Step 2   Compare present practice with this standard
- Step 3   Modify your practice to make the standard attainable
- Step 4   Repeat the process to confirm improvement

Step 1
The choice of topic is vast. Involvement by all staff concerned is important, since their future commitment is paramount. Often a topic with financial implications e.g. immunisation targets, or one in which clinical care has been questioned e.g. sudden death can be chosen. It should be relevant to the practice's needs and lead to improved patient care. The topic can be chosen from several areas e.g.

- Practice structure e.g. surgery premises, range and type of equipment, the records system and organisational systems design
- Processes e.g. examinations undertaken, prescriptions written, tests carried out, advice given
- Outcomes e.g. social functioning, psychological functioning, physical functioning and patient satisfaction

When conducting an audit a very specific question should be asked e.g. How good is our management of hypertension? An agreed standard is then determined e.g. 80% of patients with established hypertension aged 20–35 will have a diastolic pressure less than 90 mmHg within the first year of treatment.

Step 2
Data should be collected so that it can be compared to the agreed standard.

Step 3

Collecting data is only of value if a change in practice results. The practice needs to be modified so that the agreed standard is reached. This involves teamwork and delegation.

Step 4

This is widely seen as the most important stage – often called 'closing the loop' since it demonstrates if improvement is actually being achieved. Excellent introductions are available in *Making Sense of Audit* edited by Donald and Sally Irvine published by Radcliffe Medical Press Ltd and *Managing Change in Primary Care* by M Pringle *et al.*, also published by Radcliffe Medical Press Ltd.

APPENDIX 3: EVIDENCE-BASED MEDICINE

Increasingly all doctors are being asked to base their decision-making on the best available scientific evidence. Unfortunately we often find that our textbooks are out of date and there are a vast number of journals which may hold our answers. The articles in the journals will either be review articles or original studies and trials. These trials and studies are of variable quality and it is often difficult to know whether their results can be relied upon. Evidence-based medicine has been defined as 'the process of systematically finding, appraising, and using contemporaneous research findings as a basis for clinical decisions'.

The practice of evidence-based medicine involves four steps:

1. Accurate identification of the clinical question to be investigated
2. A search of the literature to select relevant articles
3. Evaluation of the evidence presented in the literature
4. Implementation of the findings in clinical practice

Each of the stages requires certain skills, and these may be assessed in the critical reading component and current awareness component of Papers 1 and 2, but also to some extent in the oral examination. For example, the clinical problem may be to decide at what level of blood pressure a 28-year-old female patient should be advised not to commence the oral contraceptive pill. This is a reasonable question but may not be answerable by reference to the literature. There may be studies which look at the risk factors for hypertension in young women on the oral contraceptive pill but no level of BP may be stated. We thus would need to modify our question so that we can actually search for the appropriate evidence.

The next stage of searching for evidence requires skills in searching literature databases e.g. Medline. This usually requires a particular search strategy commonly using key words. If the appropriate key words are not selected then insufficient evidence may be presented.

Once the appropriate articles are obtained they must then be appraised, another skill which is assessed in the MRCGP examination. Finally a judgement has to be made, based on the quality of evidence and how this answers the clinical problem.

There are a number of study designs, and they are not equal with respect to the strength of their evidence. These studies can be ranked to produce a crude hierarchy of evidence, giving more weight to studies which are less vulnerable to bias.

Hierarchy of evidence

1. Well designed randomised control trial (the gold standard)
2. Other types of trials
   a) well designed control trials without randomisation
   b) cohort (prospective study)
   c) case control (retrospective study)
3. Epidemiological observational studies
4. Opinions of respected authorities based on clinical experience, including reports of expert committees

No doctor in the future will be able to get far without understanding the principles of evidence-based medicine. It is now an established part of the clear remit of health care managers. To simplify matters, doctors and healthcare managers can now refer to authoritative reviews which have used an evidence-based approach.

APPENDIX 4: ETHICAL PROBLEM-SOLVING

Every day we make numerous ethical decisions. Some are based on well known legal or professional codes (e.g. prescribing contraception for the under 16s) but most lack such clarity (e.g. how much information do I tell the patient about the side-effects of a course of antibiotics?). The possession of a clear understanding of the principles of ethics, and how they affect management, is vital for the active practitioner and is something which is essential for the MRCGP candidate.

Ethics is the science of morals and involves:

1. The application of ethical principles on which moral values and rules are based.
2. The use of decision-making skills in applying moral principles to practical problems.

All doctors need skills to enable them to recognise dilemmas, analyse them, arrive at sound conclusions and take appropriate action. We may respond intuitively but this may be inconsistent and not the result of a thorough analysis, especially with more complex issues. If we aspire to provide the best care to our patients we need to consider the underlying fundamental ethical principles and use them whenever we have to solve problems.

Ethical decision-making, where we critically reflect upon the process of making our decisions, is especially important in certain areas:

*   On entering unfamiliar territory. New situations challenge our usual way of looking at problems and hence our decision making.
*   When faced with greater than usual personal responsibility. Such situations challenge our decision making.
*   When choosing a particular option may exclude other options, thereby having far-reaching consequences.
*   When a genuine moral dilemma exists, with painful choices having to be made between two unacceptable moral outcomes.

Fundamental ethical principles

The German philosopher Immanuel Kant argued that the concept of 'person' is fundamental to ethics. Without the concept of a person, an individual who is the bearer of rights and responsibilities, ethics cannot get started. Such individuals must always be treated as ends in themselves and this concept of a person underpins our fundamental ethical principles.

1. The principle of respect for persons
- The duty to respect the rights, autonomy and dignity of the person
- The duty to promote their well-being and autonomy
- The duty of truthfulness, honesty and sincerity

2. The principle of justice
- The duty of universal fairness or equity
- The duty to treat people as ends, never simply as means to an end
- The duty to avoid discrimination, abuse or exploitation of people on grounds of race, age, class, gender or religion

3. The principle of beneficence (or non-maleficence)
- The duty to do good and avoid doing harm to others
- The duty to the vulnerable

The concept of beneficence can be widened to encompass the duty to inform and educate, enhancing the patient's ability to continue to care for him or herself.

Ethics in context

Ethical problems do not exist in isolation, and whenever an ethical decision is under consideration it is important to be aware of the legal framework that society works under, and the professional codes which effect both the doctor and any other healthcare professionals that are working for the benefit of the patient.

The advice of the General Medical Council

The basic rules under which a doctor is licensed to practice by the GMC can be obtained from the various publications which it gives free to all doctors. There are certain standards of professional conduct and these fall into the following areas:

- Abuse of professional privileges
- Conduct derogatory to the reputation of the profession
- Personal relationships between doctors and patients
- Professional confidence, including disclosure of medical information and confidentiality
- Advertising of doctors' services
- Financial relationships between doctors and independent organisations providing clinical, diagnostic or medical advisory services
- Relationships between the medical profession and the pharmaceutical and allied industries

ETHICAL PROBLEM-SOLVING SEQUENCE

1. What is the ethical dilemma?
It is important to be as specific as possible.

2. Who is involved?
The lack of recognition that there may be multiple stakeholders involved in the dilemma often leads to difficulties in day-to-day practice. Each of the stakeholders has a vested interest and these interests must be balanced to ensure an appropriate response. For example, in rationing health care there has to be a balance between the needs of the individual and that of society.

3. Are there any laws that are applicable to the particular situation?
Any doctor who decides to practise contrary to the relevant legal framework exposes himself/herself to the wrath of the legal system and is likely to appear in court! For example, if the patient requests to 'be put out of their misery' then the doctor needs to be aware of the current laws. To proactively end the life of another person is regarded as murder.

4. Are there any professional codes (GMC) applicable to the particular situation?
A doctor who decides to ignore the guidance of the GMC is likely to appear before the Professional Conduct Committee. Extensive guidance is freely provided by the GMC.

5. Consider the three fundamental ethical principles and how they apply to the situation.

6. Make a decision!

There is often no right or wrong approach but there is a need to thoroughly and systematically consider the various options available to enable the 'best approach' to be made. It is important to consider the cost/benefit of the approach, taking into account all of the identified stakeholders.

In the MRCGP examination, marks are awarded for the PROCESS of making an ethical decision rather than the decision itself. Higher scores are obtained when candidates can demonstrate that they understand the underlying principles.

Example of Ethical Problem-solving

Carl is a 22-year-old patient with schizophrenia and has a history of violence when psychotic. He regularly defaults from his long-acting antipsychotic medication and in the last few weeks has developed increasing paranoid delusions.

His employer has noticed a change in Carl's behaviour and asks for further information about Carl's past medical history.

How do you respond?

1. What is the ethical dilemma?
Should you give confidential medical information to a third party, the employer?

2. Who is involved?
The primary duty is to the patient. Other people involved (the stakeholders) include their employer but also society, which includes family, workmates and the general population.

3. Are there any laws applicable to the particular situation?
There is no statute law of confidentiality but there is a duty of care to the patient and a breach of this could lead to civil action, with resultant damages. The Mental Health Act 1983 may be applicable when someone has severe mental illness and is a danger to themselves or others, especially if the person has no insight into their condition.

4. Are there any professional codes (GMC) applicable to the particular situation?
The GMC gives guidance on patient confidentiality and when it can exceptionally be broken.

5. Consider the three fundamental ethical principles and how they apply to the situation

- Justice and equity. This would be respected.
- Respect for the person. This principle assumes that the individual can exercise their autonomy but can be overridden if the person has a mental illness to such a degree that the person has no insight.
- Doing good versus doing harm. This duty must be balanced across all the stakeholders. There is a tension between applying this duty to the individual and the society.

6. Make a decision

In conclusion, the potential harm to society has to override the needs of the individual if that person is unable to exercise autonomy. It is important first to establish the degree of mental impairment of Carl before releasing confidential information. The doctor should always try to obtain patient consent before breaking confidentiality.

USEFUL GENERAL PRACTICE/REVISION WEBSITES

www.rcgp.org.uk – Royal College of General Practitioners

www.bmj.com – British Medical Journal

www.onmedica.net

www.doctorupdate.net

RECOMMENDED READING LIST

Audit and project work
The GP Training Handbook, third edition. Edited by Michael Hall, Declan Dwyer and Tony Lewis, Blackwell Science.

The Consultation
The Doctor's Communication Handbook, edited by Peter Tate, Radcliffe Medical Press.
The Inner Consultation, Roger Neighbour, Petroc Press.

Critical appraisal
The Pocket Guide to Critical Appraisal by Iain Crombie, BMJ publishing.
How to Read a Paper by Trisha Greenalgh, BMJ Publishing.

Practice Management
Management of General Practice by P Richard, K Low, M Whelan, OUP.
Making sense of Practice Finance by J Dean, Radcliffe Medical Press.
Making sense of the Red Book by N Ellis, J Chrisholm, I Bogle, OUP.

Ethics
Ethics: The Heart of Health Care by David Seedhouse, John Wiley.
Doctors, Dilemmas, Decisions by Ben Essex, BMJ Publishing.

Clinical topics
Excellent series in Oxford General Practice series published by OUP.
Excellent series in ABC series published by BMJ Publishing Group.

Hot topics
Hot Topics for MRCGP and General Practitioners 2nd edition. by L Newson and A Patel, PasTest.

Other revision books
MRCGP: Multiple Choice Revision Book by P Ellis, PasTest.
MRCGP Practice Papers, 3rd edition by P Ellis and R. Daniels, PasTest.
Notes for the MRCGP by K T Palmer, Blackwell Science.

INDEX

Abnormal gait 151
Alopecia 191
Asthma 190
Atrial fibrillation 182
Attendance allowance 184
Autoantibody testing 153
Autosomal recessive disorder 181

Bell's palsy 192
Blistering 135
Breast feeding 181
Breathlessness 183

Cardiac disease 128
Child development 184
Clinical trials 129
Connective tissue disorders 156
Consultation models 150
Contraception 130
Cushing's syndrome 180

Dermatosis 137, 140
Diabetic skin disease 138
Diarrhoea 142
Driving 191, 192
Drugs, in pregnancy 189

Genetic conditions 155
Genital chlamydia 183
GMS payments 152

Headaches 183, 192
Heart disease 188
Helicobacter pylori 195
Herpetic gingivostomatitis 188
Hypopigmentation 134

Infantile colic 193
Inhaler devices 146
Iron absorption 143

Jaundice 157, 181

Leg ulceration 136
Lymphocytosis 145

Macrocytosis 189
Malabsorption 181

Medication 121, 131, 132
Meniere's disease 193
Mental Health Act 158
Miscarriage 182

Nephrotic syndrome 190

Obesity 194
Onycholysis 139
Osteoporosis 141, 194

Pain relief 123
Palpitations 180
Parvovirus B19 192
PMS practices 193
Pneumonia 147
Polymyalgia rheumatica 193
Pregnancy 126
Prescriptions 191

Renal failure 121
Respiratory symptoms 127, 148, 149
Resuscitation Council 194
Rheumatoid arthritis 182

Sick certification 195
Skin blisters 180
Smoking 184, 188, 191
Systemic disease 133

Tremor 190
Tuberous sclerosis 189

Vaccinations 125, 144
Vaginal bleeding 124

Welfare benefits 154

PASTEST REVISION BOOKS

MRCGP: Multiple Choice Revision Book
P Ellis 1 901198 55 3
- Over 300 questions to reflect the current MRCGP exam
- Mixture of extended Matching, Single Best Answer and Multiple Best Answer Questions
- Subject-based book

MRCGP Practice Papers: Third edition
P Ellis 1 901198 66 9
- Revised and updated to reflect the current MRCGP exam.
- Five complete practice papers
- Each paper contains SBAs, MBAs, EMQs and Summary Completions
- Detailed teaching notes
- Comprehensive revision index

Practice Papers for the MRCGP Written Paper
R Daniels 1 901198 16 2
This new title will include all question types used in the MRCGP Written Paper
- 6 practice papers, each consisting of 12 questions with 'gold standard' answers
- the questions feature MEQ, Current Awareness and Critical Appraisal formats
- Questions accompanies by a set of suggested answers

Hot topics for MRCGP: 2nd edition
L R Newson & A Patel, 1 901198 82 0
- Over 34 sections covering 'Hot topics' in punchy note form
- Up-to-date and fully referenced to journals and studies.

DRCOG Practice Exams: MCQs and OSCEs: 2nd edition
M Dooley 1 901198 96 0
Two complete MCQ practice exams with answers and detailed explanations.

To order: For 24 hour despatch call 01565 752000 or order books safely and securely online, by shopping at our website www.pastest.co.uk